MW00881216

SWIMMING

IN

OPEN WATER

The Physiology *You Need To Know* To Stay Alive When Getting In Over Your Head

by P. Mark Fromberg, M.D.

Published in Canada by:

Open Water
RPO 29167, Okanagan Mission
Kelowna, BC Canada V1W 1X0
Website: openwaterswimbook.com
Email: mark@openwaterswimbook.com

Disclaimer

This publication was designed to provide general and educational information only regarding the subject matters covered. The author has taken reasonable precautions in the preparation of this book to provide accurate information as of the date it was written. However, the author does not take any responsibility for any errors or omissions, and specifically disclaims any liability resulting from the use or application of the information contained in this book, as it is not intended to provide individualized professional, medical, or sport coaching advice related to the unique and any specific open water swimming environment.

There are many generally known risks and challenges when undertaking open water swimming, that also vary with every individual (many are outlined in this book); therefore this book is intended to provide general guidelines only. For any specific medical or coaching advice, you are advised to consult your physician, swim coach, or sports psychologist, as indicated, prior to following any advice in this book.

Dedication

SWIMMING IN OPEN WATER: The Physiology <u>You Need To Know</u> To Stay Alive When Getting In Over Your Head is a resource dedicated to all those unsung, safety-oriented volunteers who give their time and their expertise supporting open water swim events and triathlons. They usually do so without expecting reward or recognition, and yet they share their time to help enrich their community, for the love of the sport, and to keep aspiring athletes of all ages safe while they challenge their abilities and pursue their bucket lists. Without them, so many personally enriching, health-promoting and even life changing sporting events might never occur. Always remember to say thank you to your supporters!

Motivational Quote

"All those factors out there [and in life], you can't control them, but you have to have intelligent answers to them, you have to have solutions."

- --Diana Nyad, legendary long distance swimmer, author of **Find a Way**.

Introduction

Learning to Swim as an Adult. Learning to swim as an adult was a tremendous accomplishment for me—I had been both dreading and long-avoiding this "unfinished business", before finally summoning up the courage to commit to some lessons. Like many non-swimmer adults, I had long felt overwhelmed by the many skills that I thought I would need to learn to become a successful swimmer, but was surprised how smoothly it went--after 10 step-by-step, pool-based lessons, followed by a season of participation with an adult swim club, my confidence, comfort and skills in water soared. I was finally over a mental barrier that once felt insurmountable, and felt ready to test my abilities in some open water swims, and even my first triathlon.

The Pool vs. Open Water. However, there were many differences between swimming in a pool vs. swimming in a lake or sea, and I would learn about many of them firsthand as I grew my swim experience into open water during my first summers as a newbie swimmer. And then, after a couple of years as a regular attendee at our local Masters swim club, I took interest in becoming part of the organizing committee of Kelowna's Across The Lake Swim, an event that served as a long time fundraiser for the club. It was with this organizational perspective that many important features of safety planning for the event became more obvious, and a further reminder that there were different aspects to both swimmer support and mitigating risk in the open water milieu compared to pool swimming.

And over the next decade, I was able to further my open water knowledge base by providing medical support for dozens of events—mostly triathlons and open water swims--where I would come to better understand many of the unique difficulties that competitive athletes encounter while swimming and racing. I wrote about my experiences in the first book in this series, *"Swimming In Open Water: Become Less Anxious And More Confident When Getting In Over Your Head,"* published in early 2018. For those interested, I would recommend that it should be read first, ahead of this book, given its broad introduction to open water swimming.

Deaths in the Triathlon Swim. It was also during this period (from 2000 onward) that an unusual trend in triathlons had surfaced: virtually every year there had been a few fatalities, with the clear majority of them occurring early in the race--the open water swim leg. It seemed odd that these deaths were occurring--well before dehydration, exhaustion, or overheating could be possible factors (as is often the case in marathons). It was also unsettling that the causes of these deaths were less than clear—most often defaulted to either "drowning" or "cardiac arrest"—yet these were occurring in otherwise fit, competent, athletic individuals. This trend has since been reported on several times in the last decade, with a comprehensive review recently identifying some 90 swim deaths between 1985-2016 (see Part 4, under General References). Personally, and professionally, I kept asking, what has been going on here? What are we missing? And what, if anything, can be done about it?

Knowing the Physiology. This book will try to answer these questions. While there are risks in any demanding or "extreme" sport, managing and mitigating such risks is critical to maximizing safety and enjoyment of the participants, and ultimately growing the sport. In the case of reducing swimming risks and fatalities in triathlon, understanding some common physiological responses with exposure to race conditions in open water is a key first step for both race directors and participants to mitigate risks. So read on: I hope you will find the topic of physiology in open water swimming as fascinating as I have.

Mark Fromberg, M.D.
Past President, Across The Lake Swim Society
ATLS Race Director, 2009-11
Ironman Canada Medical Director, 2010-12
Kona Ironman Medical Tent 2008-14
Kelowna Apple Triathlon Medical Director, 2010-15
Cherry Blossom Triathlon Medical Director 2014-15

Outline

As mentioned above, this book is the second in the **Swimming In Open Water** series, and serves to provide important background information only introduced in the first book (learn more about the series at openwaterswimbook.com). Although the following descriptions of medical concepts and physiological responses have been simplified to be understandable, the nature of the topics covered may nonetheless be sobering—it may even seem that swimming in open water is intolerably risky.

However, like the enjoyment of many extreme sports—whether sailing, mountaineering, rock-climbing, scuba-diving, paragliding, or auto-racing--mitigating risks in open water swimming is maximized when gaining an intimate understanding of what can go wrong and why. And, like the development of any skill, even learning to drive, it is easy to feel overwhelmed at the outset, only to realize that a logical sequence of small lessons learned will eventually accumulate and lead to mastery.

This book has 5 parts, of which the first 3 are the essence of this review:

Part 1 summarizes the many triggers that are potential physiological stressors when swimming in open water. To become a master of your open water milieu, it is important to first realize that the human body is affected by many variables commonly present in open water, each being a stressor that can potentially elicit a physiological reaction; and because these responses are potentially maladaptive, reducing their impact is key to modifying risks in open water.

Part 2 outlines these known physiological reactions, and is the core of this book. Most of these reactions can be life-threatening due to their profound effect on lung, heart, brain and/or limb function; some can develop dramatically and quickly, while others may have a more delayed effect. This section lists and describes the presumed and studied mechanisms behind these potentially adverse, physiological responses. After each of these descriptions, solutions are provided--the best recommendations and preventive strategies to minimize or eliminate each of them.

Part 3 provides a summary of the "Solutions" sections of Part 2 for easy reference, and in an appropriate checklist-like sequence. Where appropriate, there are added drills and exercises appropriate to reducing these physiological risks. To maximize open water swimming enjoyment, the goal for all participants is to be proactive, knowledgeable and prepared at all times: to accept some risks, but to responsibly manage them; to acknowledge fears, but to challenge them with a reasoned approach and alternative perspectives; to grow your knowledge base, by learning from every swimming and exercise experience (yours and others'); and to become fluent in your unique physiology and personal health, as you develop a disciplined, preventive mindset, whether young or old.

Part 4 provides some links to useful references, both in the lay press and as academic articles, many of which can be linked to as online resources.

Part 5 is an appendix that includes an acknowledgement section, and an about-the-author section. There is also an introduction to the third book in the Swimming in Open Water series.

By the time you complete this read, you should have a clear idea of how to mitigate your risks when getting in over your head; even better, your confidence in open water may have grown enough to consider coaching other newcomers to open water swimming, or to eventually become a race director of a triathlon or open water swim. And if you do, stay tuned for the third book in this series--a race director's guide to keep a mass of swimmers safe in open water.

TABLE OF CONTENTS

PART 1: The Triggers in Open Water

Introduction.

Most of us on earth live near a body of water. Whether it supplies us our drinking water, nourishes our crops, enables our sanitation systems, or feeds us with a renewable fisherman's harvest, we really cannot survive without large amounts of accessible, fresh water.

We have a more visceral connection too: The natural, timeless and untamed beauty of water—whether of a lake, a sea, or a river--constantly attracts us to its edge. We are all drawn to the interface between those superpowers of land and water—the shoreline--where the relentless surf pounding onto rocks and sand can mesmerize us as it slowly brings mountains down. And beyond the waves, the entrancing expansiveness of an ocean's sparkling surface can reach further than we can see, seeming to reach the cosmos with every sunset.

Although the power of water can make us feel small and insignificant, it nonetheless nurtures us, and, at 70%

of our body weight, it is a major part of us; the calming effect that can occur as we embrace its importance is good therapy, reminding us to stay connected to this important part of our natural world. The water is, after all, where all life forms came from, and it will be around long after we are gone.

And yet... Looking at water, or consuming water, is one thing, while actually getting into water is quite another. According to a 1998 Gallop poll, about half of Americans do not know how to swim, and are uncomfortable in the deep end of a swimming pool—and even more are fearful when in deep, open water. Perhaps this is because many of us were never properly introduced to swimming as youngsters, or at least, never had sufficient access to both playtime and lessons in water. Perhaps this is also because most of us have grown up in tamed, urban environments, where water is essentially inaccessible, and time spent in natural environments are few and far between. Perhaps we city dwellers have become too preoccupied with other activities, and have de-prioritized or even avoided this important connection to water.

Too bad.

Learning to swim as a child is, of course, one of the best ways to positively develop a lifetime relationship with water, and spending regular, recreational time in water is the best way to embrace a healthy, natural, water-based lifestyle. Unfortunately, if you haven't developed your abilities in the water by age 10-12, the odds are against you to ever succeed as an adult, even if it is just because other priorities develop and compete for limited recreational time.

Many non-swimming adults will also admit to having a bad experience in water growing up, adding a barrier to learning, and spawning any number of fears or anxieties that, without solutions, become entrenched. These may be simplistically summarized as, "If I swim in deep water, I am going to drown". Or "…die." Or "…sink to the bottom." Or "…get eaten by a shark." Or something similar. Whatever the fear, it is usually something that acknowledges a profound and growing lack of water confidence. Therefore, for non-swimming adults willing to revisit their lack of swimming confidence, a logical, systematic approach in a safe environment becomes necessary.

As it happens, there is a laundry list of factors that can contribute to the accumulation of these open water swimming fears. They are found both in the water, and in you. As you read the following list items, try them all on for size to see which ones resonate with you. Consider first the *external* variables that open water challenges you with.

The Water.

Anyone who has gone to the beach for a swim will note some obvious differences with the swimming experience in a pool. Consciously reviewing and understanding these differences is the first step in developing a solid foundation to confidence in open water.

i. First, the open water milieu is more expansive, more intimidating, more unpredictable, usually deeper, and more dynamic; it may have swells, hidden currents, and oscillating tides. It can also be affected by quickly changing weather fronts, creating rain, lightning, current, wind and/or waves. Clearly then, when going swimming in the great outdoors, proactively knowing the day's weather forecast and water conditions becomes an important safety step.

ii. Second, open water environments—lakes, reservoirs, rivers, seas, and oceans--vary more in temperature, even day to day; importantly, these bodies of water are usually significantly colder than the average swimming pool. Since the human body has several important and dramatic responses to cold, it is critically important to understand the degree of your cold exposure—both the time spent in the colder water environment, and the degrees difference between body and water temperature--when you are "out there" on an extended swim. Even in temperate summer climates, where the water temperature of a lake or ocean may be a seemingly comfortable 20-22°C, there would still be a

15°C+ difference between core body temperature and the water, which is more than enough to affect an uninsulated swimmer in various ways--especially with prolonged exposure.

iii. And third, both what is *in* the water, and what is *on* the water can provide new and significant concerns for open water swimmers. Consider swimming through a crowd of other swimmers, various types of watercraft, polluted water, or debris; being visually challenged by fog, smoke, glare, large swells, or darkness; assessing significant underwater hazards, aquatic plants and wildlife; or just getting used to the impurities or salinity of the water itself.

None of these are usually found in the pool setting. Some of these may require immediate evasive action (possibly including rescheduling your swim), some need only some increased vigilance to avoid, and some just take some getting used to. However, one or more of these variables can become a potential psychological stressor, and can become additive, potentially increasing your anxiety, and risking your ability to cope calmly and intelligently. Feeling overwhelmed with too many uncertainties is often a function of inexperience, but can lead to panic, especially when well away from immediate support or an exit point.

Clearly, these many external open water variables are already enough to affect your physiology and your psychology, for which you will need to adapt to when leaving the pool environment. But there is more--and it is all about <u>you</u>.

You.

Consider now the *internal* factors that can influence the safety of your swim: The variables *you* bring to a swim on any given day, many of which you may previously not have given a second thought.

These include your age, your overall health and previous health history; your conditioning; your experience and self-confidence in open water; your tolerance to the cold; your focus and state of mind; your level of fatigue; what medications or street drugs (including alcohol) you may have taken recently; what food or drink you have recently ingested; whether you warmed-up; your level of effort while swimming; your performance expectations on the day; any suppressed fear or anxiety that open water triggers in you; your familiarity with the day's weather forecast; the location you are swimming in; your ability to see, whether with or without goggles; your body's build and natural insulation; and what you are wearing—e.g., a wetsuit, or just a swim suit.

Given how many triggering variables there are, and how many interactions are possible, all of which can overwhelm the inexperienced swimmer and initiate physiological stresses, one may even question if anyone can feel comfortable swimming in open water.

With all these vulnerabilities evident with swimming in open water, a checklist approach may be useful to stay safe, or at least a preventive mindset that incorporates planning and foresight. As Diana Nyad suggests in her quotation at the beginning of this book, you can't totally control all these factors, but you must have intelligent answers and solutions to them--pre-thought out where possible--when you are in an uncontrolled environment, on your own, and well away from the security of solid ground and immediate rescue.

As described earlier, there have been dozens of open water swimmers that have died in open water swimming events, especially since 2000, prompting questions as to what exactly happened to these seemingly healthy, athletic individuals. In the last decade, media articles have speculated that most of these fatalities have been caused by either enlarged hearts, panic, pulmonary oedema, drowning, or most simply, heart attacks. However, as will become clear in Part 2, there is no one unifying explanation why these deaths have occurred; rather, there are several plausible mechanisms — most of which, as it turns out, involve several of the factors listed above, and are preventable once they are fully understood.

By the time you have finished this book, you will

hopefully conclude that thinking preventively is essential to the enjoyment of open water swimming. Many outdoor sports and activities use checklists or algorithms as preventive safety strategies, especially where the risks are potentially high. Similarly, many professions also use checklists--commercial pilots, surgeons, deep-sea divers, sea captains, astronauts, and civil engineers, among others--all following well-established preventive guidelines to avoid potential catastrophes. A checklist approach for open water swimmers will be presented in Part 3.

Time to sink deep into the core of this book-- Part 2.

PART 2: The Physiological Responses When Swimming in Open Water

Introduction.

Many Issues, Many Solutions. This section lists the commonest physiological reflexes that can affect people swimming in open water, some of which have been implicated in the triathlon swim deaths mentioned earlier. Given the nature of these reflexes, and how difficult they are to assess while in open water, or even posthumously, many of these reactions will remain as speculative causes of these deaths on the water. Although this section lists 18 different potential mechanisms as if they occur in isolation, in real life situations several may be at play simultaneously.

Solutions to reduce risk are provided with each discussion. A preventive checklist based on these solutions follows in Part 3.

For more background information on these mechanisms, Part 4 supplies relevant references, which are organized into subsections. Links have also been provided to most of the triathlon swimming deaths that have been reported in North American and the UK, up to the end of 2017, to allow the reader to better understand the conditions that may have contributed to each tragedy.

1. The Physiology of Breathing.

Most simply, the breathing cycle serves two vital purposes: bringing needed oxygen (O_2) into the body to metabolize your body's fuels for energy production, while also getting rid of carbon dioxide (CO_2), the waste by-product of this process. On land, the breathing cycle is all but automatic as it adapts easily to changes in exercise levels and fuel consumption. When your biochemical needs to both utilize O_2 and clear CO_2 increase, breathing rates and volumes increase proportionately, usually with minimal conscious effort.

Breathing On Automatic Pilot. The physical aspects of breathing seem almost effortless as well—at rest, (mostly) your diaphragm and (minimally) your intercostal muscles function easily to move air into your lungs, alternating with expirations that almost effortlessly fall out of your face. Even when the demands of exercise increase your respiratory rate (causing your chest wall to heave upward and outward to maximally open the chest cavity for more air movement), your body continues its effortless control of breathing. Most of the time, then, when breathing fresh air on land, these control mechanisms operate so well it is uncommon to need to ever consciously override them. It is therefore easy to take them for granted, to the point you may never feel a need to learn how they actually work.

And yet, in the water environment, in an otherwise normal healthy person, breathing control is often quickly and completely upended, especially if that person is an inexperienced swimmer. In this milieu, a cascade of destabilizing events usually follows—shortness of breath leads to anxiety, which can become life-threatening if a full panic attack sets in. What this means, essentially, is that if you cannot keep your breathing under complete control while swimming, nothing else—not your stroke mechanics, your stroke efficiency, or even your fitness—matters. **Breathing control becomes the most important swimming variable to master**—everything else is secondary, or fine-tuning. Which begs the question: How does anyone with a lifetime of normal respiratory experience so quickly lose control of basic breathing when in water?

The answer lies in learning two important aspects of the physiology of breathing, both of which become clearly apparent in swimming.

CO2, Not O2, Drives The Urge To Breathe.

First, there is an important physiological principle relevant to all swimmers that seems counterintuitive: The biochemical stimulus to change the rate and depth of breathing (such as with exercise) is primarily driven *by the build up of CO_2*, and *not* the need for O_2. So what has that got to do with losing control of breathing in water?

Since swimmers can only inhale when their face is at least partly out of the water, being in water forces you to change how and when you can breathe. The land-based, automatic drive to breathe has to be replaced with a "manual override"--to consciously control and vary the timing, rate and depth of both their inspirations and expirations, depending on the position of your mouth and nose relative to the water's surface. A new, rhythmical breathing pattern has to be created that can integrate with the swimming stroke patterns, while still being effective in balancing O_2 and CO_2 needs. Given the critical need to keep CO_2 levels low, a conscious effort is also needed to *prioritize expirations*, keeping them at least equal to inspirations in depth and duration--a task that is much easier when breathing automatically on land. For newbie swimmers, these are all new skills.

Unfortunately, inexperienced swimmers wrongly prioritize their *in*halations, thinking that their feelings of shortness of breath are because they are short of oxygen. They tend to overly initiate inhaling, while incompletely exhaling, unwittingly building up CO_2 in their lungs.

Instead, it would be much better if newbie swimmers become aware that *it is the blowing off of carbon dioxide with better (more complete) expirations that reduces the drive to breathe* (not gulping more oxygen), which, in turn, effectively reduces anxiety over breathing. The more one can *completely* exhale, the easier it is to keep your breathing rate under control, even as physical demands increase.

Exhaling In Water. The second breathing lesson that new swimmers have to learn is forced exhalation. To maintain, as closely as possible, the normal resting breathing cycle while swimming, one has to learn to exhale directly *into* water.

This does not feel normal for at least two reasons. First, when face-down in water an exhalation does not automatically "fall out of your face", as it does on land. Since water is 1000 times denser than air, it provides resistance to air entering it. An expiration has therefore to be somewhat forced, with active engagement of both chest and abdominal muscles, to get sufficient air (and specifically, enough CO_2) out of the lungs. This is a skill that has to be learned.

Secondly, forcibly exhaling all of your air into water may also feel risky. For those lacking water confidence, deliberately emptying your lungs when face down in the water creates a sense of vulnerability, and requires trust in your ability to promptly turn your head back to the surface to get enough new air in—a leap of faith that my be especially difficult in a new and unfamiliar environment. Wanting to empty your lungs may also feel wrong if you maintain the belief in prioritizing air intake (and especially O_2 intake) over exhalation.

Without being comfortable expiring into water, it is not surprising that newcomer swimmers will tend to incompletely exhale with their unbalanced breathing cycle, leading to a build up CO_2 in their lungs. A tell-tale sign of an oxygen-focussed "breath-saver" is the swimmer who creates expanded cheeks that are holding in extra air as they dive into water.

SOLUTIONS: Learning to Breathe *into* Water.

To avoid the consequences of shortness of breath and anxiety in the water environment, to keep your respiratory rate calm and controlled, some breathing adaptations are necessary, all of which keep carbon dioxide levels in the lungs (and blood stream) low.

a) Learn to Actively Balance Inspiration with Expiration. Unconsciously, at rest and even while sleeping, we tend to spend as much time expiring as inspiring—a principle that has been promoted for centuries for optimal respiratory function and deeper relaxation. And beyond keeping these phases of breathing equal, Ayervedic training in yoga has long encouraged lengthening these phases, and adding pauses in between them. Accomplished yogis can breathe as little as four times a minute, which is less than half of what an average healthy adult breathes.

In high-level sports, such as in cycling and running, many coaches also focus on keeping the inspiratory and expiratory phases approximately equal to improve performance. Oxygen uptake and CO_2 washout are optimized when inhalations and exhalations remain deep and essentially even, which maximizes breathing relaxation, while prolonging control and efficiency.

Because of both exercise demands and the need to keep breathing rates relaxed with good clearing of CO_2, swimmers would significantly benefit from breathing training, especially with extending expirations (since they take more effort). Adding pauses to breathing cycles, both before and after expiration, is an excellent confidence builder and a relaxation training technique, especially for anxiety-prone swimmers.

b) When Swimming, Become An *Active* Breather. When in water, breathing control cannot be passive: you have to be both 1) selective about timing when you breathe in (only when your mouth is at least partly above the waterline), and 2) committed to exhaling at least as much air out as you inhaled in. While such conscious control takes more effort than normal, with practice and time in the water, it gets easier, and almost as automatic as when breathing on land.

c) Get Comfortable Breathing With Force.
With inhalation during most kinds of swimming, you may only have a second to inhale a significant amount of air (usually several liters) appropriate for the swimming effort you are making. This will require inhaling through an open mouth (the nasal passages are too small to move large amounts of air), and actively using the inspiratory muscles of your chest, which lift the chest wall upward and outward to increase lung capacity. Think of it as a big, quick, forceful gulp of air.

Exhalation in water also has to be consciously forceful, especially given the ongoing need to wash out CO_2. There are two forces to generate. First, since expirations are directly into water, an increased expiratory force is required to overcome the surface resistance, and drive sufficient air out of the lungs.

When actively swimming, this should not be difficult; right after a swimmer has taken a deep, forceful breath in—after a near maximal inhalation, the stretched elastic tissues of the chest wall passively but quickly recoil, automatically squeezing air out of the lungs as the ribs start to collapse back to their resting position.

However, to get air *completely* out of the lungs, further exhalation is necessary using a different, *active* mechanism. The air still remaining in the chest (after the elastic recoil) needs to be forced out with an active contraction of both the intercostal muscles (they bring the ribs closer together, compressing the chest), and the abdominal muscles (they push the diaphragm back up into the chest cavity). Without this second generated force, lung emptying is incomplete: CO_2 will quickly build up in the lungs (and blood stream), increasing the urge to breathe even more.

d) Understand the Differences Between Diaphragmatic vs. Chest Breathing. When you are in a fully relaxed state, breathing is shallow (less than a liter of air moving) and mostly "diaphragmatic": that is, the diaphragm is the only muscle working, causing a rise and fall of the abdomen as it pulls air in and then lets it out (hence it is also called "belly breathing"). Compare this to a physically active state when the chest becomes involved, heaving visibly, and at a higher frequency than the resting state belly breathing. Chest breathing requires more effort, but gets much more air moving in and out, since it uses the many accessory muscles of the chest and neck (such as the intercostals and scalenes) to increase the size of the chest cavity. The abdominal muscles are used as well to accelerate and complete exhalations, as previously described.

In most aerobic exercise, forceful breathing is mostly initiated by chest movements, and finished with abdominal movements. The difference in swimming is that these breathing efforts have to be coordinated with the swim stroke. The best way to learn this is to build the stroke around, and secondary to, your breathing cycle (which must be established first), *and not the other way around*. To learn more about establishing a breathing cycle in water, training drills were covered in the first book in this series, *SWIMMING IN OPEN WATER: Become Less Anxious and More Confident When Getting In Over Your Head.*

e) Adapt To An Unbalanced Breathing Cycle. Since freestyle swimming breathing patterns encourage two or three arm strokes before a quick inhalation, freestyle appears to require both an inflexible (following the arm cadence) and unbalanced (quick inhale, slow exhale) breathing cycle. In the inexperienced swimmer, this adaptation from normal, "balanced" breathing patterns (when inhalation duration equals exhalation duration) can be challenging—it requires a forceful, "big gulp" inhalation within a second or less, followed by a slower, complete exhalation, drawn out over several arm-strokes—an imbalanced, asymmetric breathing cycle.

Although the ability to breathe in a large amount of air through an open mouth improves quickly with swim fitness and respiratory muscle conditioning, learning to time the prolonged expiration can be more difficult, given the need to find an optimal expiratory flow rate that will reliably get you to completely empty at the exact moment you need to breathe again. One effective way is to break your exhalation into two or three parts (coinciding with the number of arm strokes per breath—e.g., 2 parts with breathing every two strokes, or 3 parts when breathing every three strokes).

When breathing every three, the first part of your exhalation coincides with the elastic recoil of your chest, and should be effortless. It begins as soon as your face re-enters the water after the inhalation, and ends as the first of the three arm strokes is completed. Exhalation then continues with activating the chest intercostal muscles to further compact the chest capacity, and lasts approximately the duration of the second of the three arm strokes. The last part of the exhalation adds abdominal muscle use, tightening the abdomen as the diaphragm gets pushed into the chest cavity, squeezing what little air is still left in the lungs. This phase roughly coincides with the last half of the third arm-stroke.

If you are breathing every two arms strokes, the second and third phases of exhalation are combined and accelerated. If you are breathing every four or five strokes, then your exhalation pattern will become protracted, but it must always finish with a fully contracted chest followed with an abdominal and diaphragmatic push.

To be sure that your exhalation is continuous, humming a different note with each of these expiratory phases is a simple reassurance that you are continuously moving air out, and not breath-holding. It will also reduce the risk of any water entering your nose at the moment you turn your head to breathe, especially if you add a last-second snort to your humming. This provides a last push out of any remaining air, and completely clears your upper airway ahead of what will be a powerful inhalation through your mouth.

f) Commit to Staying Relaxed, Developing Flexibility. Since breath control is so critically important to sustained swimming, swimmers must remain relaxed in all their swims, and not get distracted by other anxieties that may present themselves during the swim. Arguably the best way to keep calm, while avoiding shortness of breath (and inevitably anxiety) is to keep lung carbon dioxide levels low--maintaining effective and complete exhalations, **no matter what other distractions there may be**. Many good swimmers have been known to have their breathing rhythm fall apart, even quickly, as soon as they are in either a competitive or an open water environment—their anxieties distracting them from maintaining their conscious control of complete expirations.

And finally, to become bullet-proof with breath control, it is also critical to develop flexibility in breathing patterns, particularly with expirations. Since open water swimming conditions and exercise demands can vary a lot from day to day, learning to exhale at different rates with different arm stroke patterns provides flexible options to breath control, and further adds confidence when taking on a variety of swimming conditions.

Keep CO2 levels low, and have adaptable, flexible ways to exhale as circumstances vary. These two principles must be mastered before attempting to further adapt to the many other demands of open water swimming (cold water, waves, increasing pace, sighting, wetsuits, other swimmers, etc.). Once you have mastered complete expirations, and learned to change breathing patterns—you are much less likely to be overwhelmed by the other variables described in the following sections.

2. The Cold Shock Response.

The Effects of Sudden Cold Water Exposure.
Most of us are pretty familiar with this: when we quickly
expose ourselves to total body cold, such as when
jumping into cold water, our almost instant response to
the cold is to tighten up and start breathing harder. This
reaction is your body's automatic response to the need to
preserve body temperature. Initiated by stimulation of
cold thermo-receptors in the skin, blood vessels quickly
contract and narrow in all superficial areas exposed to the
cold, otherwise known as massive vasoconstriction.
When blood vessels clamp down quickly like this, there is
an equally dramatic increase in cardiac workload, since
the peripheral resistance caused by this vasoconstriction
forces the pumping action of the heart to work much
harder. This increases oxygen demand for the heart
muscle itself, as well as for the muscles that have
tightened up and started shivering (to generate heat). And
when demand for oxygen increases, the respiratory rate
responds proportionately.

The Risk of Sudden Cold Exposure. For
someone with a heart condition or poor cardiovascular

fitness, and especially an older individual, a sudden, significant, persistent physiological trigger like this may be too much for the heart to bear. If the heart muscle is not strong enough to overcome the increased peripheral resistance, blood will back up into the lungs, causing progressive shortness of breath (medically, this is known as "congestive heart failure"). Angina may also develop--severe chest pain caused by an inadequate blood supply to these strained heart muscle tissues—and can even herald a full blown heart attack ("myocardial infarction") if blood flow to the heart muscle remains severely impaired. And each of these--cardiac strain, angina, and myocardial infarction--can also be associated with any number of cardiac arrhythmias, some of which may be lethal by themselves (more on these later).

Swimmers in open water will commonly be affected to varying degrees by the Cold Shock Response, given that open water venues are generally cooler than most pools. This is especially true in the early outdoor swimming season, when swimmers may also be unacclimatized to cold water. Since human body core temperature is normally about 37°C, it is not uncommon for open water swimmers to swim in water at least 15-20°C colder, enough of a difference to initiate the Cold Shock Response.

This cold reaction clearly makes breathing control more difficult. If a swimmer is suddenly breathing hard and feeling shortness of breath, while feeling a pounding heart rate and quickly becoming very cold—even before they start swimming--the associated anxiety, (and, for some, the progressive feeling of impending doom) can be overwhelming. Together, shortness of breath and anxiety are not good conditions for controlling inspirations and focussing on complete expirations.

SOLUTIONS: Mitigating the Risk of The Cold Shock Response.

Such a response is less dangerous and less dramatic in fitter, younger swimmers--especially those who have acclimatized to the cold (both with regular exposure to swimming in cold water, and with easing into the water on any given day). Swimmers who have higher amounts of insulation, whether as body fat or a properly fitting wetsuit, are also less likely to be adversely affected. Not surprisingly, mammals such as seals, whales, dolphins, and walruses do not have a cold shock response, due both to their built-in insulation and their acclimatization.

Acclimatize, Insulate, Ease Into It. Lessening this adverse response is straightforward: Acclimatize to cold water at every swim, primarily by *easing* into cool water. Let your feet acclimatize over a minute or two, then your hands, and then allow water to gradually enter and warm up in your wetsuit. Splash some water on any still dry, exposed areas like your face and neck. Get a sense of how fast your heart is beating and how hard you are breathing—both need to be under control before you start swimming, otherwise breath control will be very difficult from the outset.

By swimming in cool water regularly, you will soften your response to the cold, especially if you ritualize your graduated entry as described above.

Early in the season, full wetsuits should be strongly considered unless the water temperature is over 24°C. If water temperatures are under 15°C, consider double capping or using a neoprene cap—pull your cap as far over your forehead as possible. Using larger goggles can also help, since they cover more of the face. Be aware that your risks for cold shock are greatest with colder water, and if you are thin, dehydrated, older, unfit, or just not acclimatized.

Medication Effects, Other Health Conditions. Are you taking a regular medication? Some medications reduce your heart's response to the cold, and some cause excess peripheral blood flow, which accelerates heat loss. Cardiac drugs, anti-psychotics, alcohol, and antihistamines have been implicated in how well you conserve body heat. You may also be at some risk of cold sensitivity if you have hypothyroidism (an underactive thyroid gland) or have Raynaud's syndrome (excessively reduced blood flow, especially in the fingers and toes, in response to cold or emotional stress). Know your vulnerabilities—if you are not sure if any of your medications may be affecting you, or how any of your health problems may be affected by swimming in cold water, or if you are having unusual effects of being in cool or cold waters, consult a physician.

3. The Mammalian Diving Reflex.

Conserving Oxygen When Underwater.
Aquatic mammals (e.g., seals, dolphins, otters, whales, and walruses) and diving birds that stay underwater for extended periods of time utilize the diving reflex to conserve oxygen use. Humans are also known to display a strong diving reflex in infancy, although it diminishes into adulthood. However, it remains important for open water swimmers to understand this reflex, since the effects may still be significant in some circumstances.

This Reflex Begins with Your Face. When your face is quickly submerged in cold water, trigeminal nerve receptors relay this sensory information to the brain, stimulating the autonomic nervous system to spare oxygen use through several mechanisms. The degree of the effect is proportional to the coldness of the water, and it is enhanced further with breath-holding. Unlike the Cold Shock Response described earlier, it is not triggered by any of the other parts of the body contacting cold water—only the face.

The Three Main Effects of the Diving

Reflex. These mechanisms all have potentially significant consequences to swimmers in cold water:

1) A slowing of the heart rate ("bradycardia") by an average of 10-25%. This effect is noticeable within 30 seconds of cold exposure and is magnified by breath-holding, as well as swallowing or choking on cold water.

2) Decreased blood supply to the limbs ("peripheral vasoconstriction") occurs due to the constriction of the smallest blood vessels that are farthest away from the body core, which decreases oxygen usage in those tissues. The response adds to the general vasoconstriction generated by the Cold Shock Response

3) A "centralizing" shift of blood volume to the chest cavity, which is the direct result of this peripheral vasoconstriction.

Four Implications of The Diving Reflex for Swimmers in Cold Water. There are several health risks associated with the effects of this reflex:

1) Paradoxical messages to the heart. When swimming or racing in open water, this reflex slows the heart at the same time that the heart rate is ramping up (both the result of the Cold Shock Response and when starting exercise); hence the neurological and hormonal messages to the heart are therefore paradoxical, increasing the risk of a cardiac arrhythmia (more on this in the next section on Autonomic Conflict).

2) Increased risk of other abnormal, life-threatening heart rhythms. The Diving Reflex's induced slower heart rate also creates more time between heartbeats, increasing the risk of other kinds of abnormal heart rhythms to enter the cardiac electrical cycle. These are known as the "re-entrant" arrhythmias. Since breath-holding, coughing, or swallowing cold water also slow the heart rate, these are additive risks in vulnerable individuals.

3) Further work load to the heart. The increased peripheral resistance generated in the limbs by the Diving Reflex adds to the resistance provoked by the Cold Shock Response. Along with the stimulus of exercise (swimming) and any anxiety/jitters (common in pre-race swimmers and triathletes), the heart has to confront an additive cardiac load that may overwhelm susceptible (usually older) athletes: As described in the previous section, angina, congestive heart failure, or even a myocardial infarction are possible.

4) Compromised breathing. With peripheral vasoconstriction, blood pressure increases and blood volume shifts into the chest cavity. These effects can initiate fluid spilling into the lungs, ("pulmonary edema")—an effect that can cause progressive shortness of breath at a time when breathing efficiency is critical for performance.

When Is The Diving Reflex Initiated? So the question arises: How cold does the water have to be to initiate the Diving Reflex in humans? Probably less than 16°C, although, cold acclimatization, overall health, age, fitness, hydration state, and insulation may influence this estimate. Chances are, if it feels dramatically cold to you, it is cold enough to elicit a diving reflex.

SOLUTIONS: Lessening The Effect of The Diving Reflex.

First, get used to swimming in cool open water by going out into it regularly — just as you would to lessen the Cold Shock Response.

And second, recall what many Olympic swimmers do before starting their races: initially splash water on their face and neck (and body) before diving in to start a race. Walk into the open water if you can, immersing yourself gradually and feeling the coolness of the water. At the same time, wet your hands and apply them to your face and neck. If the water is particularly cold (16°C/61°F or less), you might then consider a series of short head dunks or swims of only 5-10 seconds, standing with your head out of the water in between, to acclimatize your face to the cold.

If you have any concerns, or if this cold exposure

feels in any way abnormal, check your pulse in your neck before you enter the water and again after you have acclimatized, to get a sense of how you are doing. Make note of your both your heart rate (it should not be unusually slow or fast) and its regularity (it must be regular, regardless of rate). If you have any history of heart problems (such as arrhythmias, congestive heart failure, or angina), if you are older or unfit, or if you have had any unusual physiological responses in water before, you might consider a cardiac review with your doctor prior to undertaking open water swimming—especially if you will be in colder water most of the time.

4. Autonomic Conflict.

The Two Major Neurological Control Systems. The Autonomic Nervous System is part of the body's peripheral nervous system-- it operates largely unconsciously, controlling most basic body and internal organ functions. It is comprised of two parts: the Sympathetic Nervous System, which tends to ramp things up, such as in the "fight or flight" response (described in the next section); and the Parasympathetic Nervous System, which tends to tone things down, by calming, slowing and stabilizing—it is known as the "rest and digest" response, reducing heart rate and blood pressure, while encouraging homeostatic mechanisms like digestion to flourish. An autonomic conflict arises when both of these systems are concurrently activated—analogous to having a foot on the accelerator and the brake pedal at the same time when driving a car.

How These Systems Get into Conflict. In a landmark 2012 research paper on drowning, authors Michael Tipton and Michael Shaddock reported that the most impressive autonomic conflict happens with rapid submersion in cold water, when combined with concurrent breath-holding. In this circumstance, the Cold Shock Response is initiated *sympathetically*--increasing heart rate, blood pressure and especially breathing rate (hyperventilation). This response is countered with the Diving Reflex, which is mediated *parasympathetically*— slowing the heart and breathing rates (as breath-holding does) to conserve energy and extend underwater time.

The Implications of an Autonomic Conflict. Cardiac arrhythmias can occur when the heart is concurrently being given conflicting messages, such as being both stimulated to increase heart rate, while also being suppressed to slow down heart rate. These authors also identified several other triggers that could further add conflict to these autonomic inputs to the heart. These include 1) the choking response (described in the section on Near-Drowning Reflexes), 2) the startle response (Hey RDs: don't use a noxious-sounding air horn to start an event!), 3) a large meal (see the section on Digestive Effects on Swimming), 4) several medications (see the section on Long QT Syndrome in the section on Abnormal Arrhythmias), 5) sudden and significant anger (a good reason to stay calm in open water races), and 6) hypercapnia (the build-up of carbon dioxide in the blood and body) due to poor breathing control and incomplete emptying of the lungs, discussed earlier.

Parenthetically, arrhythmias have not been reported in diving mammals. Although they have a strong Diving

Reflex, they are well-acclimatized to the cold, and therefore lack a significant Cold Shock Response--so no autonomic conflict occurs.

Although (in humans) *either* a strong *sympathetic* or *parasympathetic* stimulation of the heart can occasionally create an abnormal cardiac rhythm independently, it is when both occur simultaneously that arrhythmias are most likely to follow. Surprisingly, Tipton and Shaddock found altered cardiac rhythms in a staggering 60-80% of young, fit, and healthy volunteers, with even higher rates among less-fit individuals. Since some of these arrhythmias can potentially be lethal—e.g., ventricular tachycardia, ventricular escape rhythms, torsades de pointes, bigeminy, supraventricular ectopic beats, AV block, and atrial fibrillation--these are not rhythms you would want to be stimulating while in open water.

And there is more. The more intently researchers have looked at autonomic conflict, the worse it appears. First, since it is known that more *parasympathetic* cells predominate in the atria (the top half of the heart), while *sympathetic* innervation dominates the (lower half) ventricles, different parts of the whole heart can create conflicting electrical signals. Imagine the top part of the heart trying to slow down as the ventricles are trying to speed up—calming and exciting effects on the heart at the same time! The normal electrical pattern seen on an EKG would be torn apart with this autonomic conflict, creating the groundwork for electrical chaos.

And second, it doesn't help that the slowing effect of the Diving Reflex decreases blood flow to the cardiac muscle at the same time that more blood (and therefore oxygen) supply is needed to for the increasing demand of the ventricles. This oxygen supply/demand mismatch can put ischemic strain on the heart, increasing the risk of arrhythmia further, and increasing the risk of either cardiac "decompensation" (where the heart cannot handle the blood being supplied to it), or even a heart attack, especially in those with established coronary vessel disease.

You may wonder why potentially life-threatening cardiac issues like this don't appear or get reported more often. Fortunately, arrhythmias can, and do, spontaneously revert back to normal in the majority of cases, especially in those with healthy hearts, and who are otherwise young and fit. And given the general inability to do cardiac monitoring while swimming, many of these cold-induced arrhythmias will, for the foreseeable future, remain undetected, especially if they are transient and minimally symptomatic.

Given the many triggers of an autonomic conflict that can occur in cold water, it is clear that arrhythmias are a risk in open water swimming. Of the dozens of deaths witnessed in the swim portion of triathlon, it is fair to postulate that at least some of them may be well be the result of an autonomic conflict-induced cardiac arrhythmia. Unfortunately, arrhythmias cannot be proven post-mortem, or by most cardiac monitors while in water. Without more objective evidence, these deaths are instead most often documented as simply "cardiac arrest" or "drowning", the end result of a major arrhythmia.

SOLUTIONS: How to Avoid Cardiac Arrhythmias.

The strategy is clear: To avoid an autonomic conflict, reduce the strength of the stimuli known to provoke one.

a) The strategies to reduce the Cold Shock Response were described earlier: With every swim in cool water, ease your way into cool water, warm up the water in your wetsuit, and avoid plunging into cold water to avoid the sudden shock of the cold. Being calm and relaxed (not angry); avoid drugs, alcohol or a big meal prior to open water swimming. And focussing on blowing off CO_2 as you establish your swim will also reduce risk.

Swimming in cold water regularly with these strategies will effectively acclimatize you, blunting your responses to the cold, and reduce your risk.

b) Avoid triggering the Diving Reflex by diving into cold water, which would expose you to a sudden cold stimulusto your face. Instead, dampen the reflex when you first enter the water by splashing water onto your face and neck. As you first enter the water and start swimming, avoid breath-holding. The colder the water, the more important this strategy is. Gauge your response to the cold water on your face by how much it triggers your heart rate and your respiratory rate—if either are noticeably higher, simply wait until they have calmed down before you start swimming. Otherwise, you may lose control of your breathing very quickly, which would increase your CO_2 levels.

Race directors of open water swim events should be encouraged to avoid startling your swimmers with the blast of an air gun (a simple verbal countdown is better), as well as making sure everyone has had an opportunity to get comfortable and warmed up in the water before the event begins.

5. The "Fight or Flight" Response.

Basic Survival and the Adrenaline Rush. As an acute, total-body stress reaction, the "Fight Or Flight" Response is a basic survival instinct: it is a comprehensive neurological discharge of the Sympathetic Nervous System, unleashing a powerful adrenaline rush that primes the body to confront or flee when life is perceived to be on the line. Fortunately for most of us, such a dramatic release is only an occasional experience, since we spend most of our waking hours in a relaxed, unthreatened, homeostatic state.

Of course, adrenaline release is not an all-or-none event, nor always desperate. Even mild degrees of anxiety, such as anticipating a competitive sporting, academic, or public speaking event, can release small amounts of adrenaline, which in turn can improve focus and resolve, and even enhance outcomes.

Swimmers, too, can benefit from this anxiety, with an anticipatory adrenaline surge that would enhance performance in practice or competition. Some elite swimmers may even thrive on it, as a necessary part of the thrill of their racing experience. However, there can be stressful swimming circumstances when adrenaline release is significant and excessive, even if you are highly competitive. Many specific situations can further add to open water swimming anxiety—e.g., fear of swimming in a crowded, mass start; self-doubt of one's abilities; or worry about the water conditions of the day—these can all be additive, and build toward the feeling that you are fighting for your life. So, what happens when your stress reaction reaches a critical mass?

The Physiological Effects of Adrenaline. When someone is sufficiently stressed, their <u>Fight or Flight Response</u> triggers release of significant amounts of adrenaline. The body responds with:

· Increased blood pressure, heart rate, and stroke volume

· Increased respiratory rate and tidal volume

· Increased muscle tone and tension, improving efficiency, strength and speed

· Blood vessel dilation in your muscles to allow increased physical work

· Constricting the blood vessels in areas of the body not needed for the fight or flight, e.g., skin and intestines

· Release of the fuels--fat and glycogen (to become blood sugar)--for energy production

· Dilation of the pupils to improve vision

· Enhanced blood clotting function to reduce

blood loss

·   Increased mental attention to negative stimuli—a heightened awareness of threats

·   Increased emotional reactions (both anxiety and aggression).

The Adrenaline Rush in Open Water Swimming. How does this reflex play into open water swimming? If you are relaxed when swimming, without fear or anxiety, then it is unlikely that you will trigger these responses during your swim. However, there may be a variety of circumstances that can change your controlled state while swimming, which alone or additively provoke anxiety and therefore an adrenaline rush. Consider any of these:

1) If have not adequately warmed up, and the cold water causes you to hyperventilate even before you have reached your race pace;
2) If you get caught up in the rapid ramp up of a race (i.e., if you are pushing yourself too hard against stiff competition);
3) If in the middle of an intense effort, you miss a breath, or get struck, or run over, or pushed under by other swimmers;
4) If you get distracted by the activities of other swimmers, lose confidence in your abilities, or lose control of your breathing for any reason;
5) If the open water or swimming conditions deteriorate and become dangerous (e.g., with bigger waves or a stronger current);

6) If you become angry or encounter aggressive behaviour with another swimmer in an event;

7) Or if you suffer from the sudden onset of a medical condition (several described later) while in open water.

•

When you develop a true fear for your life, adrenaline's effects can dramatically stimulate blood pressure, cardiac contractility, heart rate, and respiratory rate. When these effects occur while swimming in open water, life-threatening cardiac events, panic and/or exhaustion can ensue.

SOLUTIONS: Avoiding the Adrenaline Rush.

Given the possible risks to significant adrenaline exposure, it is critical to keep your adrenaline and anxiety levels under control, especially when racing in an open water event. Here are 10 preventive strategies:

1) Get in a relaxed swim warm-up to acclimatize to the water;

2) In a mass start, seed yourself appropriately (position yourself off to one side, or just delay your start to avoid crowding;

3) Know your own abilities and limitations;

4) Get out of harm's way by avoiding other, faster, more aggressive swimmers;

5) Take turns wide if there is lots of swim traffic at a corner buoy;

6) Make sure your equipment (e.g., wetsuit and goggles) is familiar to you and in good working order;

7) Develop and use flexibility in your breathing cadence to avoid CO_2 build-up when doing an extended swim;

8) Know the course and the conditions (e.g., waves, wind, current, tides, rocks, hazards, creatures, boat traffic, weather forecast, and temperature) before you get into the water;

9) Have reliable and well-established alternative breathing cadences and a fall-back, alternate "recovery" stroke;

10) And always be prepared to walk away on a given day if the conditions are unsafe for you.

Staying calm in open water is always the best way to have a successful swim. Even though it may be a race, try to de-emphasize your expectations of a specific result — some of which may be out of your control anyway. Consider reframing your race as simply an event and enjoy the journey, each and every stroke. Open water swimming can even be meditative if you allow yourself to mentally relax during your swim — the ultimate way to avoid any adrenaline surges.

6. Near-Drowning Reflexes.

Choking on water. In 1985, Japanese researchers were able to record what happens to heart rate, heart rhythm, blood pressure, respiratory efforts, and consciousness immediately after water enters the trachea. Their conclusions were dramatic: choking on water is another potent *parasympathetic* trigger that slows down heart rate—a response that can occur within just seconds of aspiration (water entering the airway).

This slowing effect on the heart by choking can even stop the heart completely ("asystole"), leading to a cascade of pre-terminal events. These include a dramatic decrease in blood pressure ("hypotension"); a terminal (inadequate) breathing pattern that impairs oxygen delivery to the body; ventricular fibrillation (a chaotic, ineffective, life-threatening heart rhythm); and with all of these, an inevitable loss of consciousness. All these physiological responses would occur reflexively, *before* water has fully entered the lungs. In a swimming environment, death could quickly follow.

In open water conditions, many circumstances could

easily lead to choking on water, even in experienced swimmers in seemingly benign conditions. Missing a breath and/or inhaling water due to irregular waves or the actions of other swimmers (e.g., being struck in the face when turning to breathe) is not uncommon. The choking risk is thought to be greater in prolonged swims, since the sensitivity of the trachea to water is thought to increase with fatigue.

SOLUTIONS: Avoiding the Near-Drowning Reflex.

It should not be surprising that growing your open water swimming experience (especially with waves and mass swims) remains a primary strategy to avoid this reflex. As well, most experienced swimmers have developed and have confidence in their breathing pattern flexibility (easily changing breathing cadence to every 2, 3, 4, or 5 arm strokes as conditions dictate), should there be no air to breathe on turning the face out of the water. Experienced swimmers have also developed active, protective control of the airway using the back of the tongue and soft palate to block water from entering— these soft tissues can be quickly moved backward consciously to obstruct the airway--much like what happens passively in snoring and especially sleep apnea.

7. Commotio Cordis.

Chest Trauma can Lead to Arrhythmia.
Commotio Cordis (Latin for "disruption of the heart") is
a very unusual event initiated by something striking the
chest wall. This has been occasionally reported to occur
when struck with a baseball, hockey puck or fist. If the
blunt trauma is directly over the heart, and at a key phase
of the cardiac cycle, the cardiac rhythm can be disrupted,
initiating a potentially fatal arrhythmia. It is more likely to
occur in thinner individuals. Resuscitation of these rare
events has been poor, probably because it was
unrecognized as a cardiac event.

**A Blunt Blow to The Chest While
Swimming.** While it is not known if a trauma-related
arrhythmia has ever occurred in an open water swimming
event, that may simply be because it would have been
either unwitnessed (since it would have occurred
underwater) or unreported (the victims do not usually
survive). Nevertheless, open water swimmers—especially
lean athletes with a thin chest wall-- need to be aware that
being struck on the chest by someone's heel kick can
have lethal consequences. And this lethality is
compounded by limited rescue abilities in an open-water

setting, where timely access to a swimmer in distress is notoriously difficult.

Is Commotio Cordis an insignificant concern for open water swimmers? Possibly. However, in her 1998 book *Open Water Swimming* (on p.49), legendary endurance swimmer Penny Lee Dean outlines her experience on how competitive open water swimmers who don't like being drafted or having their feet touched may retaliate with hard heel kicks to the body. Alternately, with the rise in popularity of triathlon and mass-start open water swimming events, the close proximity of hundreds of swimmers makes for circumstances that would make such a trauma theoretically more plausible.

SOLUTIONS: How to Avoid Chest Trauma.

Since this risk arises only in group swims or mass open water starts, the definitive solution is to find some open water to swim in, while avoiding close contact with other swimmers. In open water swims, consider seeding yourself well back or off to one side, or even consider delaying your start a few seconds to avoid the heel-kicks or arm-strokes of other swimmers. When in a crowd of aggressively kicking swimmers, move away from them; avoid chest wall exposure to trauma, and/or use a slightly more protective "catch-up" stroke. When overtaking swimmers, especially breast strokers (and their whip-kick), give them a wide berth.

8. Common Abnormal Arrhythmias.

Chronic Cardiac Rhythm Disturbances. Heart rhythm disturbances can appear at any time in life, first being diagnosed even well into adulthood. Some of these can only be identified under specific conditions, and some become more common simply with aging or with new onset heart problems. The more common ones are listed below--all can appear with, or be worsened by, the increased workload or stress associated with exercise, including open water swimming.

I. Wolff-Parkinson-White Syndrome: "WPW" is a congenital (a structural abnormality you are born with) cardiac disorder that is relatively common and usually asymptomatic; it is found in about 2-4 people per 1000 population, and is more common in males. Because its symptoms may not appear until middle age, it is suspected that many adults do not know that they have it.

In WPW, there is an extra connecting electrical pathway between the atria and the ventricles in the heart that can at times "pre-excite" the ventricles to contract prematurely, leading to a rapid, but inefficient, heart rate ("tachycardia") with palpitations--followed by dizziness, weakness, and shortness of breath. The tachycardia can be provoked by exercise and, once established, can provoke various secondary arrhythmias, such as supraventricular tachycardia (SVT--a fast, but regular heart rate arising in the atria), atrial fibrillation (AF--an irregular, inefficient heart rate), and atrial flutter (an extremely fast, inefficient, but regular heart rate). Although these secondary arrhythmias may cause only intermittent symptoms, they do increase the risk of ventricular fibrillation and sudden death. The good news is that WPW is usually detectable on a routine EKG, and symptoms can be elucidated further in cardiac stress testing.

WPW in Open Water Swimming. Needless to say, becoming unusually dizzy and short of breath while swimming in open water can be disastrous, especially if the WPW pathway activates when at race pace. Being at increased risk of ventricular fibrillation while in water because of this abnormal congenital electrical pathway is potentially lethal.

SOLUTIONS: Neutralizing the WPW pathway.

If you have had recurring spells of dizziness, fainting, palpitations, or tachycardia (under any circumstances), seeing your doctor and having a routine EKG is potentially life-saving. If there are further suspicions, other investigations would be useful to confirm the diagnosis. Fortunately, there are immediate treatments available that slow down and normalize the heart rhythm, though the definitive treatment of WPW is the destruction of the abnormal electrical pathway by a procedure called radiofrequency catheter ablation.

II. The Long QT Syndrome (LQTS). This is a relatively uncommon (about 2.5% of the population) electrical disturbance of the heart that can be inherited or acquired. Medically it is referred to as a "channelopathy", as it is characterized by abnormalities of the ion channels that pass ions (such as potassium, sodium, calcium, and chloride) across the cell membranes in the process of depolarization and repolarization (the processes involved in the heart muscle's contractile functions). When these channels operate abnormally, the repolarization of the cardiac process on an EKG is prolonged (the QRS complex is the big blip that indicates the ventricular contraction and is followed by the smaller T wave, the repolarization wave), hence the name "Long QT" syndrome.

When the repolarization (electrical recovery) process is prolonged, the risk of re-entrant ventricular arrhythmias is increased (a similar risk with the Mammalian Diving Reflex); the most dangerous arrhythmia it can cause is called "torsade des pointes" (so-called because it looks like twisting up and down spikes on an EKG), a very unstable and symptomatic cardiac rhythm that usually causes dizziness, fainting, or seizures. It can quickly revert back to normal, or just as quickly lead to a fatal arrhythmia such as ventricular fibrillation.

Diagnosis of LQTS. Symptomatic, congenital LQTS is more common after age 40, and is somewhat more common in women. If you have any recurring and unexplained symptoms, or if there is any known family history of long QT syndrome, of sudden death, or of any other genetic cardiac abnormality, a cardiac assessment that includes an EKG would be necessary for a clear diagnosis.

Many External Triggers of LQTS. The majority of LQTS is, however, acquired, and not genetic. According to the Mayo Clinic, more than 50 medications are known to lengthen the QT interval (and many more are suspected): antihistamines, decongestants, anti-depressants, some classes of antibiotics (macrolides and quinolones), cocaine, diuretics, heart medications, cholesterol-lowering medications, some diabetes medications, some anti-fungals, and some antipsychotic drugs make the list.

Electrolyte imbalances can also lengthen the QT

segment--low potassium, magnesium, and calcium are common triggers that can be the result of poor nutrition, anorexia nervosa, exercise exhaustion, and even a diarrheal illness.

Previous heart disease, physical stressors such as exercise, and psychological stressors such as anger, and even loud noise can also precipitate the Long QT Syndrome in susceptible individuals. The more of these triggers present, the greater the risk of a fatal arrhythmia.

SOLUTIONS: Preventing Acquired LQTS.

If an EKG has confirmed the diagnosis, a medication review of any of your prescriptions with your doctor or pharmacist will confirm if these are possible triggers. A discontinuation plan should then usually be considered, along with a discussion of any continuing risks when swimming in open water.

Alternately, being well-nourished, avoiding discretionary over the counter medication use, and maintaining a calm demeanour with racing, swimming, or other athletic events reduces the risk of developing LQTS. If you have been ill, or if you start your event electrolyte-depleted or dehydrated, you should reconsider your participation in open water swimming for the time, until you are better.

For congenital LQTS, other treatments may be available, but ongoing risks in open water would need further discussion with a cardiologist, and would depend on other concurrent variables.

III.   Atrial   Flutter/Atrial   Fibrillation.   As implied by their name, these arrhythmias arise in the atrial part of the heart (above the ventricles), where the cardiac electrical rhythm originates; they both cause rapid heartbeats and therefore are also known as *supra-ventricular* tachycardias. They also both create a dissociated rhythm pattern from the ventricles--the contraction rate of the atria is different than the rate of the ventricles—and both are more common with aging, endurance exercise, and with heart disease.

Both can be occasional or frequent, and both are provoked by a wide variety of stressors, including electrolyte abnormalities, alcohol, thyroid disease, and stress. They are usually treated with either various medications, electrical cardioversion, or ultimately, ablation. These arrhythmias can be very symptomatic, especially with palpitations, dizziness, weakness, and an anxious feeling of impending doom. Needless to say, having an onset of either while swimming in open water can be a significant cause for concern.

Atrial Flutter. Atrial flutter can cause a dramatically increased atrial rate-- 240/440 beats a minute--which is typically two or three times the ventricular rate. At such high rates, palpitations and anxiety are common. The blood flow out of the heart is actually decreased (due to poor ventricular filling), leading to shortness of breath, light-headedness, dizziness and exercise intolerance. Because of poor cardiac output, blood can back up into the lungs — a process that defines heart failure. Atrial flutter can often degenerate into atrial fibrillation, which is different only to the extent that the rapid atrial rate is irregular and more variable than atrial flutter.

Atrial Fibrillation. Atrial fibrillation is the most common serious rhythm abnormality, with 2-3% of the Western population afflicted, a number that rises with age (about 15% of seniors over age 80 have the condition). It is also much more common in endurance athletes. It often becomes a chronic condition, and, like atrial flutter, causes similar symptoms of dizziness, weakness, anxiety and exercise intolerance—conditions that are not compatible with open water swimming. If you have any tendency of these symptoms, seeing a physician to properly diagnose your condition is critical for your safety as a swimmer in open water.

SOLUTIONS: Drugs or Surgery

Once diagnosed, treatment for atrial arrhythmias includes various rate- or rhythm-controlling medications, which, although they usually just control symptoms, may be sufficient if symptoms are uncommon. With increasing symptoms, both can be definitively treated with a procedure known as radio-frequency ablation. There are no known reliable preventive strategies; however, given the suspected triggers, avoiding potentially cardiotoxic drugs (e.g., various stimulants, even alcohol and caffeine), avoiding excessive participation in chronic prolonged endurance activities, avoiding electrolyte imbalances, maintaining a healthy weight, and remaining fit with a healthy diet may help.

9. Swim-Induced Pulmonary Edema (SIPE).

SIPE Overview. Until recently, "SIPE" (a build-up of fluid in the lungs associated with swimming) was a very unusual diagnosis, mostly occurring among commercial divers and military combat swimmers with prolonged cold water exposure. Symptomatically, SIPE usually begins with a fairly abrupt onset of shortness of breath and a cough, eventually producing pink (blood-tinged), frothy secretions; the diagnosis of SIPE is confirmed when crackling sounds are heard in the chest with a stethoscope.

With the increasing popularity of endurance swimming and triathlon, SIPE has become more common; some experts have speculated that it may be a primary contributor to the disproportionately high death rates seen in the swim portion of triathlons in recent years.

Conditions that Predispose to SIPE. Research has found that SIPE has been associated with a variety of predisposing factors: longer swims, higher intensities, colder water, a tight wetsuit, excessive swim prehydration, a lack of a swim warm-up, a history of high blood pressure, the use of anti-inflammatory medications (such as ASA), and the use of fish oil supplements. It seems to occur more often in females and thinner athletes, and is thought to occur in about 1-2% of triathletes and open water swimmers doing longer distances, at least 2km swims. Surprisingly, the condition does not seem to be associated with lung or heart disease, or even with aging.

The Physiology of SIPE. The symptoms of SIPE are the result of what happens when fluids under pressure leak from the small blood vessels in the lungs (the pulmonary capillaries), flooding the small air spaces (the alveoli) in the lungs.

On the *arterial* side of the circulation (the oxygenated blood pumped from the left ventricle to body tissues), two important processes contribute to SIPE: first, prolonged cold water immersion causes blood vessels of the limbs to shrink down (peripheral vasoconstriction), resulting in blood being shunted (redirected) into the chest and thoracic blood vessels; and second, this peripheral vasoconstriction forces the heart to pump harder (pushing blood into narrowed blood vessels requires more force), and reduces the left ventricular output (decreased stroke volume), causing blood to back up into the lungs (the pulmonary circulation), causing edema.

On the *venous* side of the circulation (the deoxygenated blood being returned to the heart and lungs), two other processes contribute to SIPE. First, due to the increased blood being shunted into the chest and then to the right side of the heart (from the cold arms and legs), the right ventricle will have *increased* stroke volume. Second, when this increased blood volume enters the pulmonary circulation (the blood vessels in the lungs,) it increases the blood pressure in the smaller arterioles (the smallest blood vessels). Under increased pressure, blood will extravasate (leak out of the blood vessels) into the alveoli (the small air sacs where oxygen and CO_2 is exchanged), interfering with the transport of oxygen and carbon dioxide.

The combination of increased *venous* pressure with increased *arterial* back pressure creates pressure on both sides of the air-filled alveoli, eventually breaking down the integrity of the barrier between the capillaries and the alveoli. Blood gets pushed into the alveoli from both directions, resulting in blood-tinged fluids collecting in the alveoli that obliterate the vital gas-exchange function of the lungs. This process results in pulmonary edema (fluid in the lungs), and is associated with a cough with frothy pink secretions, progressive shortness of breath, and a crackling sound in the chest with breathing.

Excess Hydration, ASA, and Fish Oils. Once

these SIPE inducing mechanisms are understood, it is clear how other factors can worsen the symptoms. Significant hydration prior to the event will increase the risk of SIPE; the more fluid you have on board ahead of time in cold water, the higher potential for fluid pressure to build up in the lungs.

Medicines like ASA-related drugs, which are well-known to reduce blood clotting by their platelet inhibition, can also enhance SIPE by contributing to increasing the bleeding tendency in the alveoli.

Fish oil supplements also have anti-platelet and vasodilatory effects, and therefore would also enhance the development of SIPE, by facilitating bleeding into the alveoli.

SOLUTIONS: Avoiding SIPE.

Since SIPE can also kill you, there are several important swim strategies to consider, especially if you have had a previous history of SIPE, are thin, female, and/or have a history of high blood pressure. Do not over-hydrate, especially before a cold water event. Warm up well. Do not take fish oil supplements or anti-inflammatory medications for several days prior to the swim. Consider how tight your wetsuit is. Confirm with your doctor that you do not have untreated hypertension.

And consider easing off how hard you are starting the race, especially in longer events, and especially if the water is uncomfortably cold.

Treating SIPE—Get Warm and Dry. When recognized and treated early, complete recovery of SIPE can occur within hours, especially among fit individuals, as soon as the primary triggers are removed.

Should you be at risk of, or develop the symptoms of SIPE, get out of the water immediately and then get out of your wetsuit; get yourself dry and warmed up, and get prompt medical attention if your symptoms persist. Although it is not clear if anything is more beneficial than the passage of time once warm and dry, IV diuretics and inhalers are sometimes also offered in a clinical setting to improve the lung symptoms.

10. Anxiety and Panic Attacks.

Why Open Water Swim Anxiety is Common. Surveys have suggested that half or more of adults have some level of discomfort when swimming in deep water, not surprising given how many never learn to swim as kids (in a pool or open water). In recent decades, the popularity of outdoor swimming and triathlon events has attracted many of these same adults--with limited swimming backgrounds--bringing renewed attention to open water swim anxiety.

Of course, open water swim anxiety can occur in experienced swimmers as well. Some may have had previous bad experiences in water. Others may have a lack of confidence or experience in the less predictable open water milieu. A few may simply harbour generalized anxiety as a personality trait, or feel overwhelmed by too many uncontrollable variables, especially swimming in a crowd.

Healthy Anxiety vs. Fight or Flight vs. Full-Blown Panic. Becoming increasingly vigilant while feeling mildly anxious prior to formal or competitive events is generally useful—it can improve your vigilance, safety and confidence, sharpen the mind to the challenge, and thereby improve your performance--although it can often deprive you of a good night's sleep. However, too much anxiety can be debilitating, especially when feeling threatened, or overwhelmed by too many uncertainties— what can be called "analysis paralysis". And if the anxiety escalates into a basic survival instinct, a full-blown, life-threatening panic can occur--irrational decisions, loss of breathing control, terror, and exhaustion--a dangerous mix in deep water.

The Symptoms of Panic. Panic and panic "attacks" can, of course, occur in almost any environment; they are characterized by an uncontrollable, overwhelming fear, by a feeling of loss of control, by irrational thinking, and by an impending sense of doom. Like the "Fight or Flight Response discussed previously, panic attacks are associated with a wide variety of physical symptoms, including a rapid heartbeat, and increased respiratory rate. However, they also include symptoms *not* driven by too much adrenaline: hyperventilation, sweating, tingling, numbness, choking, crying, faintness, and even a sense of altered reality, none of which are characteristic of the Fight or Flight Response.

In the context of swimmers in the open water setting, a panic attack can occur in the water, but notably, can also occur well before even entering it—even before arriving at the open water setting in some cases. Such an extreme response does not always have a rational explanation, although there are many possibilities: There are many who have had a bad experience in open water, some who are just generally anxious or worried ("highstrung"), and some who have developed a true, unshakeable fear of some aspect of open water swimming.

Anxieties May be Additive, and Become Overwhelming. Any number of open water swim anxieties may pose, by themselves, little more than a challenge to get over: A feeling of intimidation or embarrassment looking at capable, experienced competitors; being distracted by other swimmers nearby who may collide with you or want to overtake you; a lack of confidence in one's own swimming or sighting abilities; an uncertainty about a recurring injury; a wetsuit or goggles that are too tight or too loose; an apprehension over fish, wildlife or dead bodies lurking in the water; a worry over the water temperature, a current, or the waves on the water; a dislike of the weeds in the water; a feeling of claustrophobia with a mass start; a lack of confidence in the safety support on the water; a worry when not accessing important last minute instructions; or the sudden irritation of hearing the unexpected blast of an air horn. The greater any one of these cause anxiety, the easier it is to become distracted by them, enough to lose focus on purposeful, breathing control. As the number of these worries or anxieties accumulate, the easier it becomes to feel overwhelmed. And the more some of these trigger fear, the more likely a full blown panic attack can occur.

Can Panic Be Fatal? In 2011, an opinion piece[1] in the Washington Post posited that a primary contributing cause of deaths in the swim portion of triathlons may be explained by anxiety or panic attacks. What makes this theory plausible is that there are many significant legitimate stresses in open water swimming events, beyond the list just mentioned: the excitement, the adrenaline rush and competitiveness when starting a race; the crowding and chaos of mass swim starts; the lack of open water swim experience many participants have; the uncertainties of open water; the tendency to go out too hard (getting caught up in someone else's race strategy); the perceived pressure of friends, family and self-expectation; ingesting too much caffeine prior to starting; and even a poor night's sleep before the event. Although panic attacks are rarely, if ever fatal on land, the water environment is plainly more risky.

Unfortunately, for three primary reasons, we will never know for sure. Post-mortems done on swimming fatalities cannot find objective evidence of anxiety or a panic attack as a cause of death; the swimmer who could have explained what happened is no longer around to tell that side of the story; and eye-witness accounts by fellow swimmers and spectators may be minimal or non-existent. Yet, there are accounts of swimmers (even some accomplished ones) who have died in an event confiding to friends and family ahead of an event that they had been harbouring some dread or anxiety over the swim portion of a triathlon. There also a handful of swimmers who have actually survived a medical event in the water, who, in some cases, have some unique insights as to what happened to them.

SOLUTIONS: Decrease Your Swim Anxiety, and Avoid Panic.

So, to what degree do you harbour some swim anxiety? Does it occur with every open water swim, or just with competitive circumstances? Before you launch into a strategy to mitigate your anxiety, you will need to determine the roots of your anxiety—when, why or how it began, and when it occurs--and just how debilitating it is.

Having increased vigilance ahead of a training swim is normal and expected, and should be part of a pro-active safety strategy. Having *some* anxiety prior to an event is also normal and expected, as it will likely enhance your performance. However, if you have symptoms of anxiety that are not constructive, that you have to fight to contain, that you fear may overwhelm you, that associate with some of the symptoms described above, or that have adversely affected your swimming performance in the past, you may have some work to do.

Stepping up to admit your open water anxiety—first to yourself--is the most important. Unfortunately, many anxious swimmers downplay their fears to others out of embarrassment, and even avoid acknowledging their anxieties with their close friends and family. But considering that most adults harbour similar angsts, denial has no place in an open water swimmer's long term safety. Conversely, sharing your experience with others can be therapeutic, especially when hearing of other's perspectives, solutions and coping strategies.

Whether on your own, with trusted friends, or with professional help, you can potentially work through the many things that affect your swim anxiety. First, list the aspects of open water swimming that have adversely affected you. After you prioritize these, it may be useful to progressively expose and habituate to situations that would normally cause fear and avoidance, while in a safe environment or with an experienced fellow swimmer or coach.

You may need to redevelop trust in some things, such as your innate buoyancy, or your ability to relax even when you are "way out there". You may need to desensitize and reduce any negative thought distortions you have (e.g., fear of lake monsters or man-eating creatures nearby), even if that might need to include professional cognitive-behavioural counselling. Solutions to most of the common sources of potential anxiety are reviewed in the first book in this series, *Swimming in Open Water: Become Less Anxious and More Confident When Getting In Over Your Head.* Several candid accounts of open water anxiety in elite triathletes are shared, including some of their strategies for overcoming them.

Finally, if you are inherently and generally anxious, and worse in open water, you may consider: regular yoga or meditation; daily time swimming non-competitively in water, especially open, shallow water; less caffeine; better sleep; and discussing more strategies and ideas with other swimmers, professional therapists, or sports psychologists.

[1]http://www.washingtonpost.com/national/health-science/deaths-in-triathlons-may-not-be-so-mysterious-panic-attacks-may-be-to-blame/2011/10/24/gIQA70NrKN_story.html]

11. Caffeine and Associated Stimulants.

"Ergogenic" Caffeine is Everywhere. Caffeine has long been recognized as both a quick-acting (within 15-45 minutes of ingestion) stimulant and an addictive substance. Its use is ubiquitous in the Western world--in coffee, tea, and many soft drinks and, more recently, in "energy drinks". Among its many physiological effects, there is consistent scientific evidence that caffeine enhances physical performance--it is indeed "ergogenic"-- particularly for endurance sports, regardless of what fluid, gel, or pill it is in. Although the dose and timing prior to exercise has varied considerably in research--doses from 1-6mg per kg of body weight, given from 1-3 hours prior to exercise--there appears to be a reliable dose response curve that varies primarily with the degree of an individual's regular caffeine exposure. This is not surprising, given that caffeine sensitivity and tolerance varies widely among individuals.

And Now, Energy Drinks Too. In the last 10 years, sales of energy drinks —caffeinated beverages marketed to young adults seeking an "edge" in their activities — have skyrocketed. Products like Monster, Red Bull, Redline, and 5-hour Energy Shot have been the major players in this market. Many of these also include high levels of sugar among other enhancements, such as guarana, ginseng, gingko, carnitine, and taurine, as well as other amino acids. Of particular interest is guarana extract, a natural extract from the plant <u>Paullinia cupana</u>, the seeds of which are known to contain the highest natural dose of caffeine in the world (40-80mg of caffeine per gram, which is 4-8x more concentrated than coffee). This extract also contains other naturally occurring stimulants, such as theophylline and theobromine.

So, while the caffeine added to these drinks is up to 150 mg in a 500 mL can, it is only the beginning of the story. With the addition of 5-10 grams of guarana (a typical amount in a can of these drinks), a total dose of nearly 500 mg of caffeine in a single can of energy drink (one serving) can be reached — much higher than a standard cup of coffee (50–100 mg caffeine) or a can of cola (40–60 mg), and significantly higher than the accepted safe total <u>daily</u> dose of caffeine for adults (400 mg).

The Effects of Overconsumption of Caffeine.

Numerous toxic effects on brain, gastrointestinal, muscle, and cardiac tissue have been described with overconsumption of caffeine. The most common are irritability and anxiety (brain); nausea, vomiting, and abdominal pain (gut); tremor, twitching, and rigidity (muscle); increased heart rate, increased blood pressure, increased ectopic heart beats, and increased irregular rhythms (heart). The severity of these varies with the level of caffeine sensitivity of the individual. Some of the cardiac effects can become intractable, and some are lethal. Energy drinks have been reported to unmask some cardiac conditions, such as the Long QT syndrome (discussed previously), and the Brugada Syndrome (another genetically inherited channelopathy-- more common in males of Asian descent).

Until recently, death by pure caffeine overdose has been rare. However, with the introduction of energy drinks, several deaths have been associated with caffeine from these sources. Most have been thought to be the result of either an arrhythmia, or a myocardial infarction. It is unclear how much these deaths have been purely the result of the very high doses of caffeine in these drinks, whether alcohol, concurrent exercise or other drugs taken concurrently have also contributed, or whether other active ingredients in these products can also be implicated.

Caffeine and Open Water Swimming. So, what does caffeine ingestion have to do with swimming in open water? Given the previous discussions on autonomic responses to exercise and cold water, adding an unnecessary stimulant may require some second thought; however, this would depend on how much extra you might be taking in beyond your regular intake, as well as your developed tolerance to caffeine. If you are significantly dependent on caffeine, your regular morning dose may even settle you down. Otherwise, a significant dose of caffeine may add to any situational anxiety affecting you at the outset of the swim. And for most coffee drinkers, a strong need to urinate within an hour or less of ingestion may add a progressive discomfort to a long distance swim—although relieving oneself while swimming is probably a more common strategy than is acknowledged.

SOLUTIONS: No Added caffeine, No Energy Drinks.

Regarding caffeine intake for open water swimmers, less is probably better, given the many known cardiac effects of cold water immersion already discussed. If you have habituated to a daily caffeine intake, it is unlikely that supplementing this consumption will add any performance benefit without potentially adding risk.

Regarding energy drinks, given the added ingredients they contain, most of which have little evidence to support their use (conversely, a few have been associated with deaths in otherwise healthy young adults), prudence suggests particular caution in the use of an energy drink prior to an open water swim. Ignore the marketing hype for these products—the benefits are generally overstated, while the risks are acknowledged only in the fine print.

12. The Digestive Effects on Swimming.

"Don't Swim Right After Eating!" Sound familiar? We have probably all heard as kids this old parental advice--to not go swimming for at least an hour after eating, due to the presumed risk of cramps and/or drowning. This advice has even been documented in Boy Scouts' literature as far back as 1908!

What historical event this advice was based on remains obscure — perhaps there was once a child that drowned jumping into water after eating a meal, initiating this well-intended, but anecdotal piece of advice. But is there any substance to this? And what about this cramping? Are we talking muscle cramps, or stomach cramps? A quick Internet search can find strong opinions both supporting and refuting any significant risk of swimming after eating. So what should we advise swimmers regarding an eating strategy before an open water swimming event? As you might expect, there are some grey zones here, but there are indeed some physiological realities to consider.

The Physiology of Blood Shunting. The first important normal body function to understand relating to digestion and exercise relates to the concept of "blood shunting"--the physiological process that automatically shifts the blood flow from one area of the body to another, depending on metabolic need. For example, when the digestive process is well underway (usually within the first hour after eating a meal), blood flow to, and metabolism in, the gut is increased dramatically to support the significant demands of digestion. This blood supply is diverted from other body tissues that are relatively inactive, such as from the skin, muscles, some internal organs, and even the brain.

Recall your last big meal—a Thanksgiving dinner perhaps. Within an hour or so after eating a large amount of food, it is common to feel disinclined to exercise or to concentrate on anything—even feeling sleepy, or preferring to lie down to rest, at least until the digestive process has subsided. You may even notice feeling cooler skin or an unexpected chill (especially going into a cooler environment) after eating, signs that blood flow has moved away from underutilized tissues to support gastrointestinal (GI) functions.

Most people do not appreciate that the process of digestion is a very demanding, energy expending activity. Since it requires a significant amount of oxygen consumption, an increased blood supply is needed, and is redirected to the GI system by the shunting process.

Once underway, digestion is like two other processes--fighting a major illness or recovering from a significant injury—these all shunt blood from the body musculature, inducing cessation of activities and physical rest.

Conversely, increasing exercise demands will also initiate blood shunting, but in this case, away from the digestive system. When we are at rest, blood flow to muscles is quite sluggish, while most blood flow continues to maintain all of your working organs, including your GI tract especially the brain. If any new physical activity is introduced and sustained, the body responds over several minutes with a suite of changes to support the new muscular metabolic needs, and that includes moving blood flow away from the gut and other organs. This shunting process is easiest when there is minimal digestion taking place.

So, what happens when there are dual demands for blood supply—increasing physical activities while actively digesting a meal? Or more specifically, if digestion is well underway, how much is athletic performance impaired by inadequate blood supply caused by shunting? The answer is a question of degrees, of course. How much blood is "stolen" by the GI system from the musculature after a meal depends on:

a) How big the meal is (the bigger the meal, the larger and longer the shunting process);

b) How nutrient dense the meal is (with more nutrient density, and the lower water content, the longer the digestive period and the longer shunting is needed);

c) What proportion macronutrients (fats, proteins or carbs) it contains (proteins and fats digest slower than simple carbohydrates, while fiber—which is not absorbed--prolongs the digestive process);

d) The duration of time after the meal was eaten before exercise (the longer the time or the smaller the meal, the more likely the digestive process has completed);

e) How fast the meal was eaten (eating more slowly protracts the digestive period, but may lower the degree of shunting);

f) The level of physical activity before eating (activity causes shunting to working muscles, and will tend to decrease appetite, and resist supporting digestion by shunting to the gut);

g) And even how old, fit, or healthy the individual is (general health and fitness positively affects the efficiency of digestion and the shunting process).

•

h) Anxiety of any kind will tend to suppress both appetite and shunting to the gut, as described in the Fight of Fight response.

Digesting and Exercising Concurrently?

Essentially, when your body is fully in digestive mode, it cannot easily, also send a large blood supply to the musculature to support exercise demands, whether swimming, or anything else. Should you insist on trying to do both, your autonomic control system will first prefer to maintain the first activity, whether that is digestion, or exercise, since there is not enough blood in your circulation to support both.

If you have just eaten a substantive meal, and then try to initiate significant aerobic exercise before digestion is complete, your body will resist you, since the blood flow needed to fully support both activities will be compromised. Athletes (including swimmers) may feel dizzy, or light-headed (the brain's blood supply is decreased); gastrointestinal upset (stomach cramps, pain, nausea, bloating, and even vomiting) can also occur if gastric emptying and the digestive process are impaired due to inadequate blood supply; muscular weakness, and coordination may also be noticeable for the same reason. In the open water environment, these are conditions that impair performance and even put a swimmer at risk. Moral of the story: don't have a big meal before swimming in open water —at the very least, you won't feel very good, and at worst, you may revitalize your mother's worst fears and the urban myth of why you shouldn't swim after a meal.

SOLUTIONS: Eating Less Before Exercise.

However, many athletes do eat before exercise as a form of a calorie boost for an endurance event or workout, and they can do it safely if a few conditions are met:

a) The amount of food should be small, especially if it is ingested within an hour of any exercise;

b) The food should be easily digestible, so as not to unleash the full shunting process — gels, bananas, liquid calories (such as blended drinks), and sugared drinks would qualify;

c) The timing of anything more than a snack should precede an endurance event by two hours or more, and should be easily digestible even then (unless anxiety precludes any appetite, in which case, do not eat).

Eating During Exercise. For longer endurance events (greater than 1.5-2 hours), athletes may be inclined to take in calories <u>during</u> the event, as they deplete their glycogen supplies (the stored form of glucose in muscle and liver tissue). Studies in endurance athletes have shown that there is an upper limit at which athletes can absorb water and nutrients while exercising, given the shunting of blood supply away from the gut to active muscles. This limit decreases with higher levels of effort and with progressive dehydration in longer and hotter events. In these cases, the gut is progressively impaired from absorbing anything—even water will be vomited back up in extreme cases.

Before reaching this point, nutrient absorption can reach up to about 60-70 grams of simple carbohydrate per hour, if it is in liquid form, given in small doses, and facilitated with the presence of sodium in the drink. The nutritional strategies for longer endurance events, including swims, will need to be individualized.

Exercise on an Empty Stomach. For open water swimmers who commonly train and race in the morning, most can sustain their energy levels for as much as two hours without eating anything upon rising, relying on nutritional stores (both fats and glycogen from the previous day's meals. Having a completely empty stomach while swimming or exercising will also minimize any risk of a blood shunting conflict. Other swimmers may prefer to eat some small amount of simple carbohydrate within an hour of exercise; perhaps little more than a piece of fruit, some carb-based hydration, or some other easily digestible food.

Since we all have different physiologies, and we do different kinds of exercise at different intensities and durations, every athlete will need to experiment with their pre- and during exercise needs. For the open water swimmer, especially with shorter swims (less than 2 hours in length), eating and drinking within an hour of the event should be kept to a minimum — since abdominal discomfort, dizziness, and weakness are not symptoms you want to be dealing with well away from solid ground.

Hydration Needs for Open Water Swimmers. Maintaining hydration in swimming is not as important in shorter open water swims (<1 ½ hours) since fluid losses per hour in cool water is never as high as in biking or running. Given the risk of SIPE (discussed earlier) with over hydration in long open water swims in cold water, caution regarding hydration (both pre-event and during the event) is advised.

To clarify your fluid losses in swimming, get an accurate weight of yourself (most digital scales today can measure within a tenth of a pound) before and then immediately after a swim workout, without drinking or urinating between weighings. You will find that the weight lost (your fluid losses) over an hour is usually well under one pound (less than ½ liter of fluid loss), much less than doing the same experiment after a running or cycling workout. Such fluid losses are small and are unlikely to impair performance, and can wait, to be easily replaced after swimming.

For longer events, especially multisport events, a scheduled hydration plan should be considered, but will depend on sweat rate, air and water temperatures, wind, and variations in nutritional strategies. Such replacement is therefore highly individualized, and should be planned with a certified coach as necessary.

13. Repetitive Strain Injuries.

Common Swimming Injuries. Due to its non-weight-bearing nature, swimming is generally pretty easy on the body—injuries more often occur in land-based sports where greater forces on joints can be more easily generated. When swimming injuries do occur, they most often affect overuse areas. Of these, repetitive strain injuries to the shoulders are easily the most common (regardless of stroke); less commonly, the knee and hip can be become aggravated in the breast-stroke whip-kick; and occasionally, the low back is strained with a dolphin kick.

Muscle spasms and cramps together comprise another category of common swimming injury. Most commonly, calf cramps are known to occur in a variety of circumstances, associating with cold water swims, prolonged swims, hard kicking, excessive stretching, wall push-offs (hard plantar-flexion), dehydration, electrolyte imbalance, and even excess caffeine intake.

Other traumatic injuries, even head injuries, are rarely reported, but may occur if a swimmer is hit by watercraft or thrown by wave action onto hard surfaces—e.g., underwater rocks or coral, a dock, a pilon or the hull of a boat. Cuts or abrasions when scraping or scrambling over rocks or coral can also occasionally be significant enough to require urgent medical assessment.

Causes of Rotator Cuff Injuries. Shoulder injuries in open water swimmers most often involve the "rotator cuff", a group of four small muscles that stabilize and rotate the upper arm. These injuries are most often the result of poor stroke mechanics, where the larger shoulder muscles are off-loading too much workload onto these smaller support muscles. Restrictive wetsuits, excess use of hand paddles, poor warm up, or the "Rule of Toos": swimming too long, too fast, too often—are also often implicated in the development of a rotator cuff injury. Unfortunately, once established, these injuries can persist for many months.

Given the importance of the shoulder in swimming propulsion, developing an acute shoulder injury is more problematic in open water than in a pool, since it would almost certainly interfere with a prompt and safe return to shore.

SOLUTIONS: Assessment, Treatment and Prevention.

The many causes, diagnostic tests, and treatments of

shoulder and rotator cuff injuries is beyond the scope of this book, but a sports medicine assessment with a qualified professional can elicit patterns of pain, weakness, guarding, and decreased range of movement, as part of the process to develop a working diagnosis. Such an examination would be warranted if these symptoms are troubling, continuing, or worsening despite rest and modified activities. Once diagnosed, a search for a possible cause should begin with a review of recent provoking activities, followed by a mechanical assessment of the arm stroke by a qualified swim coach, which may reveal telling asymmetries, often best revealed with video. Ignoring increasing symptoms, or pushing through an acute or persisting shoulder pain is most often a recipe for a chronic injury.

A second common source of shoulder pain in open water swimmers is associated with wetsuit use, especially if there is tightness or restriction over the shoulder. If a swimmer has no problems when not wearing a wetsuit, but only with wearing a wetsuit, then the solutions are straightforward:

Change wetsuit size or brand, try a sleeveless wetsuit, or simply create more redundancy of the neoprene around the shoulders when pulling up the sleeves. Always test your shoulder range of motion once your wetsuit is on, and before you get into the water—if your movements are restrictive or painful, adjust the neoprene.

Once water gets into the suit, the neoprene will tend to adjust itself to minimize stresses; however, if shoulder symptoms persist or worsen, consider the alternative strategies.

Acute Injury While in Open Water. Depending on what has happened to you, generally the first goals are to limit any further danger of injury, arrest any significant bleeding, stretch out a cramp, or simply localize your injury, while ascertaining that your breathing is still under total control. If your symptoms are not improving with a short period of rest, and significant enough to impair further swimming, getting to safety is the next most important goal. If there is on the water support available to you, hail their attention in any way you can for assistance.

Alternately, getting back to land can be done by swimming (slowly) with a one armed stroke, by choosing an alternate, non-aggravating stroke (breast stroke, side stroke, or back stroke), or just using a kick as primary propulsion, with rests as needed. Alternately, if unable to swim without pain, it is important to retain a calm demeanour despite your injury, to avoid panic, and to find a comfortable resting posture or recovery stroke, such as a back float or treading water while summoning and awaiting support craft. In many cases, repeated short rests can keep symptoms under control and allow the resumption of easy swimming.

Muscle spasms or cramps (commonly of the calf) afflict some swimmers more than others, and can be sudden, excruciating and frightening when they occur in deep, open water without any nearby support. However, with the benefit of the buoyancy provided with a wetsuit, a swimmer can roll onto their back then grab and dorsiflex their foot to counter the spasm of their calf. Once the spasm has passed, less kicking is about the only strategy available while "out there", unless there is supportive watercraft nearby.

14.

Hypothermia/Hyperthermia.

Body Heat Loss or Gain in Water. Because water is much more dense than air, the thermal conductivity of water is also much higher than air. Calm cold water conducts heat away from the body 20-25 times more efficiently than still air does, a difference that increases when the water is moving.

The effect of swimming in warm water is similar but in reverse, where the combination of the heat of the water and the metabolic heat generated by the swimmer can result in a net gain of core body temperature.

When core body temperature drops 2°C or more, the effect is called hypothermia; when it increases by the same amount, the effect is called hyperthermia. Both are potentially lethal.

Physiological Changes in Hypothermia. Hypothermia is recognized once your body core temperature drops below 35°C (normal is 36.5-37.5°C); it can be life-threatening if the core temperature drops further. At its earliest stages, shivering increases and skin is pale due to decreased blood supply, while lips, ears, fingers and toes may turn blue. As the core temperature decreases   further:

a) Shivering stops (to conserve energy);

b) Speech becomes slurred, thinking becomes sluggish and incoherent;

c) Confusion and irrational behaviour increases;

d) Semi-consciousness and obtundation are progressive;

e) Physical incapacitation progresses with stiff movements, stumbling and muscle cramping, while coordinated movements become severely impaired;

f) Multiple physiological changes occur (decreased heart rate, increased blood pressure, decreased circulation, and increasing cardiac irritability and strain all increase the risk of death in progressive hypothermia).

Risk Factors for Hypothermia. In virtually all of the world's open water, water temperatures are significantly lower than normal human body core temperature. To stay safe and healthy, open water swimmers will therefore have to protect their core from the cold, much more so than if they are in air of the same temperature. The strength of this defence against the cold is dependent on:

a) Just how cold the water is (the difference (in °C or °F) between water and body temperature);

b) How cold the air temperature is;

c) Just how well your body is insulated against the cold (with either body fat or a wetsuit),;

d) How well your body is adapted to handle the cold;

e) How vigorous your exercise/work activities are in the water (heat generation);

•

f) How fit and how old you are;

g) How long your exposure to cold water is, and;

h) How much the water is moving or turning over next to your skin.

Most hypothermia victims are male. Men generally have less body fat (younger males especially so), and although they can also generate more metabolic heat with a greater muscle mass, they will also lose it faster, increasing their risk of hypothermia. Men are also more often doing prolonged activities in cold water, whether in a work environment, deep sea diving, doing triathlons, or simply participating in risky behaviours. The risk of hypothermia also increases with alcohol intake, and with increasing age.

Fortunately, open water heat losses can be

significantly reduced (by about 90%) when wearing a wetsuit, which can provide dual insular layers--created both by the small bubbles of entrapped gas in the neoprene, and by the water trapped and warmed inside the wetsuit.

SOLUTIONS: Steps To Avoid Hypothermia.

Know The Water Temperature. The most potent risk factor to be aware of to avoid hypothermia is water temperature.

To provide some reference points, lakes, seas, oceans, and rivers that people usually swim in can vary widely from 10°C or less to 25°C or more, a range of about 20°C. Comfortable swimming temperatures, such as in recreational swimming pools, are set at about 26–28°C, which is quite similar to the seasonal water temperature variation of the ocean temperatures of the Hawaiian Islands (25°-28°C). Temperatures of 28°–30°C+ are seen in some tropical environments, and are often used in more leisure pool environments--for babies, young children, and the elderly. Hot tubs are several degrees warmer than that, about 35-40°C.

Most open water temperatures between 20-25°C are generally well tolerated even without a wetsuit, especially if the air temperature is as least as high and without significant wind. However, as water temperatures dip below 20°C, and especially below 15°C, wetsuit use becomes increasingly necessary to withstand the effects of the cold. At these lower water temperatures, tolerance to cold is also affected by the presence of wind, the air temperature, how much the water is moving, and the warming effects of sunshine.

Although water temperatures in a lake or ocean is not readily available, it is easy to bring along a pool thermometer to clarify your thermal risk ahead of your swim. Depending on where you live, there may be also accessible government websites or even some sailing club websites that reliably report water temperatures of local bodies of water.

Assessing Body Core Temperature. To understand your individual response to cold water, the other important temperature measure for open water swimmers is body core temperature. Unfortunately, taking this measure is not quite as practical, since it requires use of a rectal thermometer. Using ear, forehead, or oral measures of temperature are especially useless in the open water swimmer, since they reflect the temperature of the water the swimmer is in, and not the swimmer's core temperature.

However, most observers can still estimate how hypothermic someone is by simply assessing their speech and their movements. In rough terms, diminishing coordinated movements and mental clarity are noticeable below 35°C, and are obvious below 34°C. Progressive obtundation and declining consciousness follow as body core temperatures drop further. These symptoms should prompt emergency medical support.

To avoid developing hypothermia while swimming in open water, consider these steps:

a) Take a pool thermometer with you to get a good idea of the water temperature. Your tolerance to any measured temperature can then be anticipated and better understood.

b) Unless the water is comfortably over 22°C, using a well-fitted wetsuit is strongly recommended for most open water swims, especially if you are thin, as it will insulate most of your body surface while providing the safety of extra floatation.

c) When the water is cold (such as 16°C or less), proportionately limit your swim time to less than an hour, even with wetsuit use, unless you are experienced and knowledgeable about your tolerance to colder water temperatures.

d) Do not swim alone when swimming in cold water, or, at least, have nearby and capable support, on shore or on the water. Should you develop symptoms suggestive of decreasing core temperature, it is important that someone who knows you can objectively observe and assess your behaviour for signs of hypothermia, and initiate appropriate and prompt rewarming techniques as necessary.

e) To learn about your tolerance to cold water, assess any symptoms you may have after all of your swims, such as shivering, slurred speech, stiff hands, or being uncoordinated when walking or trying to remove your wetsuit, and correlate that to the water temperature and the time you spent in the water.

f) Get out of your wetsuit and swimsuit as soon as you can after have exiting the water. While the wetsuit will keep you warm and protected from any cool breezes, your wet bathing suit will continue to cause you to shiver until you are out of it, towelled off, and have put on dry clothes.

g) Make sure you are coherent, coordinated, and warmed up before getting into your car to drive home.

h) If you are still feeling cold after drying off, consider outside warming with a warm shower or bath, a hot tub, or even with hot water bottles placed strategically over core areas (e.g., armpits, torso, abdomen, and/or groin). Add internal warming with hot chocolate or tea (you may want to initially avoid the higher caffeine content of coffee).

i) If you are visibly sluggish, mentally incoherent, semi-conscious, and/or your movements are slow and poorly coordinated, you will need continued support, with observation or possibly even hospital assessment, where rectal body temperature measurement would be part of the initial examination. Treatment of severe cases of hypothermia (these patients are usually unconscious) includes a gradual rewarming process, starting with the core first, to avoid the rush of cold blood from the limbs to an irritable heart vulnerable to arrhythmia.

Hyperthermia. Although wetsuits generally provide several safety factors for open water swimming, and can reduce heat loss in cool water by an estimated 90%, many open water swim and triathlon events either do not allow, or discourage, wetsuit use above 22°C. Wearing a wetsuit at these temperatures can increase the risk of *hyper*thermia (an increase in body core temperature) which has its own risks. After 26 year old American Fran Crippen died in 2010, just 500 meters from the end of the finale of the FINA 10K World Cup Open Water Series near Dubai (the water temperature was 31°C, and the air was even hotter), recommendations were made to put an upper limit to how much heat swimmers can tolerate safely, even without a wetsuit. Today, no open water swim race can occur in waters above 31°C (87.8°F) or in a combined air and water temperature above 63°C (145.4°F).

Physiological Changes in Hyperthermia. Hyperthermia is defined by core temperatures reaching 40°C or more. This heat stress is the result of either *internal* metabolism (such as is generated by intense exercise, febrile illness, and/or a poor sweat response), or *external* heat (such as immersion in hot water or air), or a combination of both (such as in the Crippen case). Hyperthermia occurs when the body's capacity to off-load the heat accumulated is exceeded.

Symptoms of heat accumulation often begin with headache, fatigue, nausea, weakness and dizziness. As body temperature rises further, confusion, poor coordination, clamminess, muscle cramps, rapid heart rate, fainting, and loss of consciousness can follow. Irreversible brain damage and death can occur quickly after.

Another potential risk of hyperthermia for swimmers is excess time spent in a hot tub or sauna before or after a swim, one reason that most of these have time limits in public settings.

SOLUTIONS: Avoid Overheating, Timely Cooling.

To avoid hyperthermia, then, avoid spending too much time in hot water, and in gear that retains body heat, such as a wetsuit or swim-cap.

To treat hyperthermia successfully, it must be recognized early, and treated aggressively. Hyperthermia is a medical emergency, and must be corrected with *immediate* total body cooling—with the use of an ice-bath if possible, even before transport to a hospital, since brain and tissue damage can occur quickly and become irreversible if treatment is delayed. If the victim is still conscious, offering cool fluids with electrolytes to drink will provide internal coolng and help counter the dehydration and mineral imbalances that are usually associated with overheating and exhaustion.

15. Acute Illness.

So, How Are You? Feeling a hundred percent? **Are you ever?** On any given day, your performance, whether at work or play, and whether physical or mental, can be significantly impaired by concurrent health issues. Recent surgery, recent injury, or a recent start on new medications can affect you. Being hung-over, or having flu symptoms, stomach upset, or drunk, or depressed, or jet lagged, or congested with seasonal allergies or cold symptoms can also profoundly affect your athletic or academic performance. These are all common events in our everyday lives, and yet all can add stress and risk to almost any experience—including open water swimming.

So, How Are You—Really? Swimming when injured, unwell, or under the influence may not only impair performance, but may also fatigue you prematurely, affect your judgment, increase your risk of hypo- or hyperthermia, and undermine your breathing control. Since several of these consequences may appear concurrently, the risk of ongoing health issues while swimming in open water can easily spiral out of control, especially when they increase your time and effort in the water.

Despite these concerns, swimmers (and other athletes) are often known to ignore their possible impairments, choosing to "push through them," especially if there is peer pressure to perform, coaching pressure to maintain a workout schedule, or just a personal and dogged determination to believe in oneself to overcome any adversity. For swimmers, this may be fine if you are testing your abilities safely, by staying within yourself, in a safe environment. But are you are willing to truncate a longer or competitive swim if things continue to feel limiting? Are you able to control your increased risks despite pressures not to?

SOLUTIONS: Can You Say No?

To commit to a true distance open water swim, there remains a determined need to call a spade a spade—to stay within one's capabilities, and to recognize when it is not your day, even if it happens to be an important event or race day. If you are unsure of your capabilities based on any of these variables, consider getting some objective advice, perhaps from a coach, fellow swimmer, or a physician, before putting yourself at unnecessary risk. It takes courage to say no, especially to peers, coaches or followers, but you must never cede control of your decision to participate in a given event to someone who is less likely to know your skills and current circumstances. Just remember that tomorrow is a new day, and that no single sporting day should ever be more important than an excess risk to health and safety. Consider reframing your decision-making process as simply an objective weighing of the variables of the day: your abilities and potential benefits vs. the precariousness and significance of the risks—is this a gamble or a well-controlled risk?

Introducing "The Stupid Line". There is often a fine line between a smart risk vs. a stupid risk—or alternately, between a calculated, understood risk, vs. an ill-advised gamble, and such divisions commonly occur in daily life and in virtually every sport. And what is ill-advised for one person may be a simple challenge for someone else. In 1994, the Canadian Injury Prevention Foundation launched the concept of "the stupid line", which was intended to help young adults consider carefully their risk-taking behaviour—whether it was diving off a cliff, trying new street drugs, drinking and driving, skiing a double diamond black ski run. Regardless of your age, you must ask yourself if you have crossed *your* stupid line: are the potential consequences of your actions reasonably certain and controlled—or not?

Any open water swim can also present this way--as a choice between a well-controlled risk vs. a questionable choice. How you feel on a given day, combined with your abilities in open water will be stacked up against how challenging the swim is on that day—how cold it is, how long the time and distance of the swim is, how much current, wave or wind to contend with, and how much support you have—is this a controlled risk or a questionable gamble? Saying no to a given swim is not a sign of weakness, but rather, of strength and courage to make a tough call, often in the face of alternate (and sometimes biased) opinions. Each of us has our own "stupid line", and it is only us that can determine whether we are crossing it.

16. Heart Attacks.

Straining the Heart. Although all physically demanding sporting events put some degree of strain on the heart, such a stress is generally thought to be health-promoting, enhancing cardiac efficiency while improving general health and fitness, especially with repeated and controlled exposure. However, when exercise strain to the heart is extreme, and/or possibly associated with other risk factors--smoking, aging, a sedentary lifestyle, chronic illness (e.g., previous heart problems, diabetes, or chronic lung disease), panic or anxiety, dehydration, or overheating--the risk of permanent heart damage--a "heart attack"--is significantly elevated.

The Physiology of a Heart Attack. So, what differentiates a healthy strain from a stress that permanently damages the heart? Like any muscle, the heart works harder during exercise--it beats more frequently and more forcefully, increasing the cardiac output (and therefore oxygen delivery) by as much as 6 times the resting rate. To manage increased and sustained workloads, the heart itself needs oxygen via a reliable blood supply, provided by healthy, unobstructed coronary arteries (the oxygen-carrying blood vessels around the heart). If even one of these arteries is narrowed (such as with age-related atherosclerosis), the perfusion of blood to the heart muscle is progressively impaired, creating "coronary insufficiency". With even mild increases in activity, such narrowed arteries often provoke chest pain ("angina"). Although angina usually settles with rest, it is a sign of significant coronary obstruction that usually mandates urgent intervention, either with stenting or bypass surgery.

Should a narrowed artery become completely obstructed with a blood clot—a "coronary thrombosis"-- a part of the heart muscle is deprived of oxygen. If this problem is not rectified quickly in a hospital with drugs that can break up the clot, some heart tissue will die--this is known as a "myocardial infarction" (MI). For those who survive this life-threatening event (about half do not), the dead tissue will become a non-functional, scarred area of the heart muscle, and will permanently affect the heart's pumping efficiency and ultimately the body's exercise tolerance.

The potential degree of injury to the heart does not stop there. With greater losses of viable heart tissue (usually the result of multiple coronary vessels compromised or obstructed), comes increasing cardiac dysfunction, both in the form of impaired electrical control of the heart, as well as the effects of having less functional cardiac muscle. Once the heart is so damaged that it cannot pump blood out faster than the rate blood is received, "congestive heart failure" develops--blood backs up into the lungs, causing progressive shortness of breath. And if the contractile function of the heart is so weak that the body's organs and tissues cannot be adequately supplied with oxygen, (especially the brain and the heart itself), death eventually ensues.

Another Probable Cause Of Many Heart Attacks. Damage to the heart muscle can also be caused by the electrical control of the heart. Under normal circumstances, the heart has a well-orchestrated pattern of electrical depolarization's that begin spontaneously at a structure known as the sino-atrial node in the right atrium (one of the two upper heart chambers); these depolarizations cause the heart's muscle cells to contract, helping to move blood out of the atria and then into the ventricles (the lower heart chambers), from where blood is pumped either into the lungs to pick up oxygen, or into the general circulation to deliver oxygen to all body tissues.

Unfortunately, various cardiac arrhythmias (abnormal heart electrical patterns previously described) can dramatically impair this efficient passage of blood through both the heart and the coronary blood vessels. When these occur in while exercising, the heart muscle can again be profoundly affected by oxygen deprivation, leading to coronary insufficiency, angina, infarction and even death. Thus the common term "heart attack" can be the result of either electrical or vascular pathology;

both can damage or ultimately stop the heart, which is known as a cardiac arrest.

Cardiac Arrest in Sport. Heart attacks and cardiac deaths are known to occasionally occur in several demanding sports—in rugby, soccer, basketball, wrestling, among others--in otherwise healthy young males. They have also long been known to more often affect older active males—the "weekend warriors", who may have more sporadic activity levels, concurrent health problems, and less healthy diets.

In studies of marathon-related deaths, death rates have varied considerably--from one in 75,000 to one in 400,000 participants—and are in fact, comparable to many other less demanding, every-day activities. On autopsy, most of these victims have been found to have some established heart disease that was previously undiagnosed, despite significant previous participation in running. Most marathon-related deaths have occurred near the end of a race or shortly afterward.

It remains intriguing that in the demanding sport of triathlon, most of the cardiac deaths have paradoxically, occurred early in the race--in the first leg, the swim-portion--well before exhaustion, dehydration, or overheating might have become a contributor to the cardiac arrest.

In most of those autopsied, a true myocardial infarction has rarely been found; and while there has often been evidence of varying atherosclerotic disease, more than half or the victims did not have any clinically relevant, structural heart disease finding.

Unfortunately, as has been described in the previous sections, significant rhythm disturbances of the heart can and do cause death during intense activities like open water swimming and triathlons, and, loosely, have also come to be called "heart attacks." However, since autopsies cannot show any evidence of the electrical rhythm disturbance, the pathology reports cannot definitively state "arrhythmia" as a cause of death. Instead, the authors of these reports often simply record "cardiac arrest"—which is technically true, but falls short of explaining exactly why the heart stopped. "Cardiac arrest" and "drowning" remain the most frequently cited official cause of death in those athletes who were not autopsied.

SOLUTIONS: Avoiding A Heart Attack in Open Water.

Should you ever suffer some kind of life-threatening event while swimming in open water, getting prompt help and getting quickly out of the water are usually critical steps to long term survival. Swimming with a personal swim buoy can help keep you afloat, and enhance your visibility for potential rescuers. Preplanning your safety before your swim can also be critical, especially in extended open water swims.

Regarding prevention, there remains considerable discussion of the merits of cardiac screening prior to the undertaking of any competitive endurance sport, and at what age such screening should be initiated, given that thousands of physical examinations and expensive tests that would have to be done for each potential life saved. Conversely, it has also been argued that undertaking a sedentary lifestyle is also a cardiac risk factor, and would therefore also demand similar screening!

Nevertheless, a previous history or a family history of sudden death, heart disease, arrhythmia, poor physical fitness, or age over 40 should all more strongly justify a comprehensive medical and cardiac review prior to undertaking competitive open water swimming. Talk to your doctor about any concerns or anxieties you may have. Then find a fitness activity that you can safely do and build from, such as swimming, since the risk of pursuing fitness to health and quality of life is without exception a lesser risk than settling passively into a sedentary lifestyle.

17. Wildlife in Open Water

Ever since the release of the blockbuster movie "Jaws" in 1975, the unspoken fear for many open water swimmers is what potentially harmful creatures are lurking in the waters beneath them. These fears are only compounded when familiarity of, or experience with, these creatures and their tendencies are unknown. It is clear though, that the contents of every environment is different: Tropical seas are different from northern seas; tropical fresh water areas cannot be compared to northern lakes and rivers.

Although various kinds of fish, diving mammals, birds, jellyfish, crocodiles, turtles, parasites and bacteria are all potential risks (immediate or delayed) to the wellbeing of an open water swimmer, a discussion of each of these is beyond the scope of this book. However, the information you will need is not far away.

SOLUTIONS: Get Educated

If you are unfamiliar with what potentially dangerous fauna and flora is in a body of water you are interested in swimming in, or if there are hidden or dangerous rocks, rip currents, waves, or tides, seek guidance from the locals, especially swimmers and others who spend time on the water, who will be able to answer your questions. Chances are if they are not keen on swimming in it, you shouldn't be either! If their counsel is unavailable to you, read what you can about the area. Being proactively well-informed remains your best strategy to keep yourself safe in unfamiliar open waters.

18. The Factors Affecting Buoyancy.

The Physics of Buoyancy. When swimming in varied open water settings, understanding the variables that affect your buoyancy can be critical for water safety, personal swim confidence, and even race strategy. To understand buoyancy is simply to understand the concept of density—of you as a body in water, and of the water itself.

More than 2,200 years ago, Archimedes had his "Eureka" moment in a bathtub when he discovered this enduring principle:

> "Any object, wholly or partially submerged in a fluid, is buoyed up by a force equal to the weight of the fluid displaced by the object."

An example may clarify this physics principle. If an object weighing 100Kg displaces a volume of water that, when weighed, would be 80Kg, then there is a net difference of 20Kg; thus, the object is more dense than the fluid it is in, and will sink with gravity. Interestingly, due to this net difference, this object's apparent weight in water will feel easier to lift while in water. Alternately, if an object is less dense than the fluid it is in, the water's greater density will create buoyant forces on the object, causing it to float.

To understand the importance of buoyancy in open water swimming, consider the density of the different body tissues of a swimmer, and the density of the water, neither of which are constant.

The Body's Constituents: Fat, Muscle, Blood, Bone, and Air. Since the human body is 60-65% water, the majority of the body has essentially the same density as the water it is in, so this part of the body would not sink or float. Since fat is known to be about 10% less dense than water, a varying proportion of the body will improve floatation (individual body fat percentages, range from 5% to 35%+). Women, in general, have 5-10% more body fat than men do, so they would be more likely to float.

Muscle and blood tends to be about 5% more dense than water, and bones somewhat more than that. Since men tend to have more muscle mass, more blood mass, and higher bone density, men have more likely to have denser bodies than women, and therefore are less likely to float.

Finally, there are parts of the body filled with air

(mostly in the lungs and connected air passages) that also contribute to buoyancy. Since competitive swimmers are well known to have larger total lung volumes due to their training than non-swimmers (as much as 20–30% higher), it follows that regular swim training will improve buoyancy. And yet this buoyancy is dynamic: Although most people would float in both fresh and salt water if their lungs were full, the regular act of breathing means that swimmer buoyancy varies with the breathing cycle as they swim.

You can add to your buoyancy by wearing a wetsuit. As a material, neoprene is about 1/6 the density of water, can improve a swimmer's buoyancy by about 3% or more, depending on the thickness of the suit. A full wetsuit can also decrease drag in the water, improving swim times by about 3-5%. Thinner (denser) swimmers would have the greatest benefits from wearing a wetsuit.

The Density of Water. The mineral content of water is the other important variable affecting the buoyancy of open water swimmers. That humans can float more easily in salt water than in fresh has been known at least since Biblical times--salt water contains dissolved minerals, its increased density providing a stronger upward force (buoyancy) on any object, such as a swimmer. Although the ability to float would be obvious swimming in the Dead Sea, where the water weighs 24% more per unit volume, it is still noticeable with the seeming small difference in density measured in most oceans, where water weighs only about 2.5% more per unit volume than fresh water. In denser water, swimmers can generally swim faster, especially in a wetsuit, since they float higher in the water (by 2.5%), with better body position, while arm-strokes can pull better with denser (thicker) water.

SOLUTIONS: What To Do To Stay Afloat.

Knowing your general buoyancy tendencies will be based on your body composition, the water density, and whether you are wearing a wetsuit. It will help you to strategize the safety of your swim, anticipate how hard you may need to work in your swim to stay afloat, and may even help you reduce any swim anxiety you have in open water. Thin, muscular males swimming without a wetsuit in fresh water would have the least buoyancy, and therefore the most difficulty keeping a head out of water, and therefore the highest risk of anxiety; they would, incidentally, also be at highest risk of hypothermia, all factors to consider for a thin male before an extended swim cooler fresh water.

Some important differences in buoyancy between fresh and salt water have long been known. In a 1977 study on human body buoyancy in 98 men, authors E.R. Donoghue and S.C. Minnigerode reported that, while all floated in both fresh and salt water with their lungs full, only 7% would float in fresh water with their lungs empty, while 69% would float in salt water with their lungs empty. This is a critical point: these male swimmers were almost 10 times more likely to be floating in salt water than in fresh water when their lungs were empty. Pretty clearly, then, swimming in salt water is safer, less work to stay afloat, and therefore less stressful, since you are much more likely to be floating under any circumstances. And since about 2.5% more of your body is above the water line in salt water than in fresh, supporters and potential rescuers would be slightly more easily able to both track you and find you, should you need the support.

Working With The Distribution of Your Buoyancy. Given that body tissues have different densities, it is also important to appreciate that these tissues are not symmetrically distributed, and therefore may affect your swimming ability in open water. The parts of you that would more easily float tend to occupy the middle and/or upper half of your body--Fatty tissues are usually preferentially stored in the central and upper torso, while air-filled structures (the lungs) are clearly in the chest. Conversely, the denser tissues that would more likely sink—muscle and bone—are more diffusely distributed, although the large volume of the lower limbs are disproportionately well known to sink, due to their high muscle and bone content.

Without a conscious effort then, body position while swimming would not, naturally, be very streamlined—the upper body floats, while the lower body sinks—although, on the positive side, it would enhance a safe, heads up position for breathing. To compensate, accomplished swimmers develop a more efficient, streamlined position, with two strategies: a sufficient kick to keep the dense legs at the surface (this is easier in a wetsuit), and a determined effort to swim "downhill", with a lowered head position. With optimal body position comes optimal efficiency and swim speed, less fatigue, and less time in the water, all of which makes for a safer swim.

PART 3: Staying Alive in Open Water—The Summary

(a) Introduction.

If you have managed to read this far, you may wonder if swimming in cold, open water is even worth the many risks so far described. However, there is risk in virtually everything you do—even walking down the street has risk—so it may be fairer to suggest that, for open water swimmers particularly, most risks are to be first recognized, and then weighed, then mitigated and managed. The following description puts the risk "solutions" from Part 2, into a practical sequence.

(b) Before You Swim Your First Stroke.

Before you start swimming in open water, or start any other exercise program—and particularly if you are older, deconditioned, have a family history of sudden death, have joint problems, significant injuries, lung conditions, cardiac conditions, a history of anxiety or panic attacks, or a history of seizures, see your doctor to get any of these potential red flags medically cleared first. A few tests may be in order, including blood tests, a chest x-ray, pulmonary function testing, cardiac screening and cardiac stress testing. Your doctor may also suggest a sports medicine or physiotherapy assessment for any physical limitations you may be bringing to your desire to swim.

There are also some secondary medical concerns-- affecting your tolerance to, or endurance in cold water exposure--that would also deserve discussion with your doctor. These might include excessive thinness, cold sensitivity, thyroid disease, Raynaud's Syndrome or a history of musculoskeletal injury. If you have a smoking history, or are on any medications, including supplements, ask your prescribing doctor if they would adversely affect cold water sensitivity or exercise tolerance.

(c) Before You Start Swimming In Open Water.

Before you transition to open water swimming, you should develop confidence, competence, and fitness in the safety and comfort of a pool. If necessary, get swimming lessons to improve your swimming skills and experience while working on your endurance and water confidence. Learning some open water skills, like "recovery" strokes, pop-up sighting, and breathing frequency flexibility, can all be learned in the pool. Knowing how to take your pulse while swimming (using the carotid pulse in the neck is best), and what a normal, regular pulse feels like are also beneficial for self-assessment, should you develop an arrhythmia while swimming.

(d) Before Your First Open Water Entry.

Unless you are normally swimming in warm water (over 22°C), you should start your open water swimming season with the insulation and floatation provided by a well-fitted wetsuit. The goggles you choose should be relatively new and seal well, and have tinted, mirrored or polarizing lenses with an anti-fog treatment for the outdoor environment. Swim caps should be made of silicone (thicker, and more insulating) as opposed to latex, and can be doubled up for even better head insulation, especially in colder waters. Invest in a pool thermometer to bring along to test cooler waters, especially early in the season.

When swimming in open water for the first time, go with experienced open water swimmers, and enter a familiar and relatively warm body of water, devoid of currents, riptides, significant waves, windy conditions, boat traffic or other hazards. Focus on staying calm and relaxed in anticipating your swim, especially if you have had anxiety problems in the past. Prioritize the development of an easy, sustainable breathing cadence. To avoid feeling overwhelmed, remind yourself to stay within your capabilities and know your limitations--and look at your swim as solo event, and not as a race.

Given that there are more than a dozen new variables in the open water environment, some of which are weather dependent, develop awareness of a swim-day's weather forecast, and take an active interest in how open water swimming is different than pool swimming. Be sure to ask of your experienced colleagues questions that relate to some of these new challenges, and to know your risks before you expose yourself to them. How cold is the water? How long will we be in cold water? Should I be wearing a wetsuit? How deep is the water? Can you safely stand in any part of the swim? Any hazards, boats, weeds, fish, or wildlife expected in the water? How do you swim in waves? Where can we dry off, change and warm up after the swim? Where can I safely put my valuables and my car keys while I swim?

Be sure that you have brought everything you need—your wetsuit, swim cap(s), towel, goggles (perhaps an extra pair), and warm clothes--and you have a rewarming strategy planned if it is cold. Being well rested, without signs of illness, stress, anger or anxiety, will also reduce several of the risks described in Part 2. Avoid overeating and discretionary uses of OTC medications, caffeine, energy drinks, alcohol, or supplements (unless specifically prescribed by a physician), prior to swimming in open water. To reduce the risk of SIPE, avoid overhydrating before a long swim in colder water, and if possible, do not use ASA or fish oil supplements during the open water swimming season. Make sure your wetsuit is comfortable, and not especially tight.

On any given day, whether based on the conditions of the water, or how you are feeling, have the courage to walk away if either feels unsafe for you. Don't cross your "Stupid Line"—where a calculated, acceptable risk becomes an ill-advised risk.

(e) Entering Open Water.

To control the Cold Shock Response, ease into cool water—even if you are wearing a wetsuit. The colder the water, the longer this adjustment might take. In a wetsuit, you will sequentially feel the cold on your bare feet, your hands, your low back (as water creeps through the zipper), your upper back, and then your neck and face as you gradually immerse yourself. If at any point you are breathing hard, you are progressing too fast—do not continue further until your breathing returns to normal, which should happen as the water in your wetsuit warms up. The more you swim in open waters, the more easily and quickly you will be able acclimatize to the cold.

To control the Mammalian Diving Reflex, splash water onto your face and neck *before* diving into cold water, especially when the water is 16°C or less. You might try a few strokes, alternating with breaststroke, or just stop and stand up, to get your face back out of the water if it feels too cold for you. If uncertain how you are responding to the cold, take your carotid pulse in your neck—it should have a regular rhythm and be between 70-100 beats per minute. If it is either higher or lower, do not start swimming until your heart rate has returned to this normal level.

If both of the above reflexes are minimized, the risk

of an Autonomic Conflict between them is also small, especially in warmer water. You can take your pulse again after you have entered the water, if you note any unusual symptoms—such as a slow heart rate, dizziness or weakness.

After you have successfully immersed yourself, spend some time warming up with some easy swimming. Assure yourself that your shoulders feel relaxed when reaching your arm-stroke out in front of you, and adjust your wetsuit as necessary.   And most importantly, establish your breathing pattern, with sustained, and full expirations to blow off CO_2.   Vary your breathing cadence to re-establish your comfort with changing your inspirations from 2-6 arm-strokes, without breath holding or becoming short of breath.

Make sure your goggles are clear and seal well. Practice some easy sighting, and start looking for the landmarks or buoys that you will need to remember during your swim.

When swimming in group training or racing events (especially mass starts) in open water, always seed yourself appropriately—to minimize collisions or the likelihood of being run over by faster swimmers. Find a small piece of open water to call your own, a space to stay calm and focus on developing your stroke and breathing patterns, while avoiding significant body contact with other swimmers, which can be troublesome and stressful.

(f) Swimming in Open Water.

Once your swim is safely underway, without other swimmers crowding you, your early swim should continue to focus on establishing sustained expirations into the water to keep CO_2 levels low and breathing rate under control. Do not focus on speed too early! Your breathing rate should start slowly, with breathing every 4-6 strokes as you ramp up to a sustainable race pace where your breathing cadence will become more frequent (usually 2-3 strokes) after 100-200 meters of swimming. Use humming if necessary to establish your expirations.

Feel the rhythm of any significant wave action that may be present. Let that rhythm determine your stroke frequency, and adjust your breathing to one side if necessary. As your stroke and sighting frequency become rhythmic, and as other sounds disappear as you increasingly notice only on the lapping sounds of the watery milieu you are in, you may sense the rhythmic and meditative aspect of open water swimming. Occasionally you may need to adjust your course, to stay away from other swimmers' arm-strokes and kicks, to avoid unnecessary chest or face trauma, or accidental choking on water, but your goal is to find the rhythm that is all your own.

If you become short of breath during your swim, or

develop a frothy pink-tinged cough after swimming in cold water (the symptoms of SIPE), call it a day--get out of the water as quickly as possible to strip off your wetsuit and to warm up, and seek medical attention if necessary.

To reduce the risk of hypothermia in the early open water swim season, take the water temperature before each swim. Limit your time in cold water when it is below 16°C, and do not swim alone. Be sure that your group is well aware of the early symptoms of hypothermia, since you may not be a reliable judge of your own symptoms. Swim in open water regularly to acclimatize to cool water swimming, and correlate your tolerance to the cold with the actual water temperature.

If while swimming, you are feeling any unexpected feelings of chest discomfort, take your pulse to assess any rhythm irregularities or palpitations. If you are feeling anxious at any point, reflect on what may be triggering anxiety in you while you swim, and take the steps necessary to reduce these triggers. If you are naturally anxious when swimming in open water, consider using a personal swim buoy (Check out Amazon for a "Swim Buddy", or at getaswimbuddy.com).

(g) Getting Out Of Open Water.

After long endurance swims, you may note sudden dizziness when standing up at the end of your swim. This is a normal reflex (called postural hypotension) that occurs in normal people changing position from horizontal to vertical too quickly, although it tends to be more noticeable when swimming, since blood has been shunted to working muscles while exercising, leaving the brain briefly vulnerable to a loss of blood pressure when standing. To avoid this, stand slowly, in deep water after some easy breaststroke (so your head is up slightly), and when taking the first steps, keep your head down, close to heart level to minimize the effect.

Once you are walking safely, proceed to dry off completely once out of open water, and get into warm, dry clothes. You should be comfortably warm and mentally coherent before driving home. If you are still cold and shivering, consider a warm shower or bath or hot tub, along with warm drinks, such as tea or hot chocolate, to return to normal temperature.

If you are a keen student of the open water experience, you may consider logging each of your swims—the water temperature, the conditions, any problems you might have had with your equipment, the conditions, or with your stroke—to develop your personal open water experience.

Summary

Well, I hope you learned a few things. This book was intended to provide background information and solutions (in Part 2), followed by an organized summary (in Part 3) of most of the important physiological issues facing open water swimmers. Will any medical screening test reliably eliminate all risks? Nope. But given the many medical problems that could contribute to problems in open water, your unique concerns about your health risks should be discussed with your doctor some of which can be mitigated with appropriate screening.

It is to be understood that swimming in open water can never be risk free—that each of us has to take responsibility for our health and manage our risks on a day-to-day basis—to dispassionately assess your own conditions of the day along with those on the water, to fairly decide what is a reasonable, vs. an ill-advised, swim. As you grow your understanding of the physiological underpinnings of open water safety, you can build your own training strategies and solidly further your open water skills and confidence.

To add further depth to the topics covered, the next section of this book provides you with lots of reference information from the scientific literature, the news coverage of the many athletes who have died in an open water swim, and the ongoing narrative in the press on the possible causes of deaths in the swim portion of triathlon. I hope these links can further embellish what you have already learned by reading this book.

If there are any physiological factors missing in Part 2, or any issues that could be expanded upon, please email your constructive feedback to mark@openwaterswimbook.com, so that the next edition can be even better. And if you found this book otherwise useful to your open water swimming training, please consider providing your honest review on the Amazon web page where you bought this book.

Your partner in open water,

P. Mark Fromberg, M.D.

mark@openwaterswimbook.com

PART 4: Selected References

General References on Deaths in Open Water Swimming

2017: Death and Cardiac Arrest in U.S. Triathlon Participants, 1985 to 2016. Harris KM, C
Cresswell LL, Hass TS, et al. Ann Intern Med. Doi:10.7326/M17-0847 19 Sept 2017.

2017: Preventing Drowning: An Implementation Guide. Geneva: World Health Organization; 2017. Licence: CC BY-NC-SA 3.0 IGO. ISBN 978-92-4-151193-3

2016: Revisiting The Triathlon Death Rate. Alexis Sobel fits. Undark July 14, 2016.

https://undark.org/2016/07/14/triathlon-death-rate-competition-endurance-sport/

2016: Why do so many middle-aged men die during ironman competitions? Samantha Allen, The Daily Beast, May 24, 2016. https://www.thedailybeast.com/why-do-so-many-middle-aged-men-die-during-ironman-competitions

2016: Enlarged Hearts May Be To Blame For Triathlon Swim Deaths. Susan Lacke, Triathlete, Sept 17, 2016. http://www.triathlete.com/2016/09/news/enlarged-hearts-may-blame-triathlon-swim-deaths_137106

2016: Deaths in triathletes: immersion pulmonary oedema as a possible cause. Moon RE, Martina SD, Peacher DF, Kraus WE. BMJ Open Sport & Exercise Medicine vol 2: 1 2016 http://bmjopensem.bmj.com/content/2/1/e000146

2015: Triathlon Swim Deaths. Dressendorfer R. Current Sports Medicine Reports: May/June 2015 - Volume 14 - Issue 3 - p 151–152 doi: 10.1249/JSR.0000000000000142

2014: Are Triathletes Really Dying of Heart Attacks? Brian Alexander, November 2, 2014 Outside Online. https://www.outsideonline.com/1926956/are-triathletes-really-dying-heart-attacks

2013: Fatal Arrhythmias in Open Water Swimming: What is the Mechanism? Larry Cresswell, Athlete's Heart Blog, March 10, 2013
http://www.athletesheart.org/2013/03/fatal-arrhythmias-in-open-water/

2013: Triathlon Fatalities: 2013 in Review. Larry Cresswell, Athlete's Heart Blog. December 30, 2013.
http://www.athletesheart.org/2013/12/triathlon-fatalities-2013-in-review/

2013: Trouble beneath the surface. Bonnie Ford ESPN October 18, 2013
http://www.espn.com/espn/feature/story/_/id/9838319/trouble-surface

2012: USA Triathlon Fatality Incidents Study. L Cresswell et al, USA Triathlon, Oct 25, 2012.
https://www.teamusa.org/USA-Triathlon/News/Articles-and-Releases/2012/October/25/102512-Medical-Panel-Report

2011: Deaths in triathlons may not be so mysterious; panic attacks may be to blame. David Brown, Washington Post November 14, 2011

2011: Why is Swimming the Most Deadly Leg of a Triathlon? Scientific American, Larry Greenemeier. August 9, 2011.

https://www.scientificamerican.com/article/triathlon-death-swimming/

2010: Sudden Death During the Triathlon. **Kevin M. Harris, MD; Jason T. Henry, BA; Eric Rohman, BA;** et al **Tammy S. Haas, RN; Barry J. Maron, MD. JAMA. April 7,** 2010. 303(13): 1255-1257. doi: 10.1001/jama.2010.368
https://jamanetwork.com/journals/jama/fullarticle/185622

2009: Warning over Triathlon Death Rate. Jeremy Laurance, The Independent. May 25, 2009.
https://www.independent.co.uk/life-style/health-and-families/health-news/warning-over-triathlon-death-rate-1690626.html?cmp=ilc-n

Individual Reported Swim Deaths in Triathlon and Open Water Swimmers

2017:
https://www.thesun.co.uk/news/4195147/man-dies-trying-to-swim-english-channel/ (44 yr old male)

https://www.straitstimes.com/sport/triathlete-dies-in-swim-leg-of-relay (42 yr old male)

www.washingtontimes.com/news/2017/dec/20/man-dies-after-losing-consciousness-during-triathl/ (75 yr old male)

http://www.scmp.com/news/hong-kong/community/article/2116469/man-66-drowns-during-hong-kong-triathlon-event-lantau (66 yr old male)

http://abc13.com/news/local-athlete-dies-during-ironman-in-the-woodlands/1903630/ (54 yr old male)

2016:

http://newschannel9.com/news/local/wife-of-racer-who-died-in-ironman-703-he-expressed-concern-with-the-swim (51 yr old male)

http://www.startribune.com/man-56-dies-during-rochester-triathlon/383555901/ (56 yr old male)

https://saskatoon.ctvnews.ca/saskatoon-woman-dies-of-heart-attack-during-b-c-triathlon-1.2883931 (57 yr old woman)

https://www.theguardian.com/sport/2016/aug/28/endurance-athlete-nick-thomas-dies-swim-english-channel (45 yr old man)

https://www.houstonchronicle.com/neighborhood/woodlands/news/article/Family-bewildered-by-death-of-fit-27-year-old-9218487.php (27 yr old male)

2015:

https://www.theguardian.com/uk-news/2015/aug/31/first-time-triathlete-paul-gallihawkfound-dead-kent (34 yr old male)

http://www.dailycamera.com/news/boulder/ci_286
23765/despite-ironman-boulder-athletes-death-experts-
say-triathlon (40 yr old male)

https://www.bloomberg.com/news/articles/2015-
04-02/canaccord-ceo-dies-from-complications-tied-to-
hawaii-triathlon (52 yr old male)

2014:

http://www.nbc-
2.com/story/24427268/competitor-dies-during-hits-
triathlon-in-naples (57 yr old male)

http://edmontonjournal.com/news/local-
news/triathlete-dies-after-heart-attack-at-edmonton-race
(59 yr old male)

https://www.ajc.com/news/suwanee-man-dies-
during-triathlon/Xtkx6Fr4ejwz1bKnQS5M2I/ (68 yr old
man)

2013:

https://www.usatoday.com/story/sports/olympics/
2013/05/15/swimming-deaths-trouble-triathlon-
officials/2164793/ (50 yr old woman)

https://patch.com/california/redondobeach/son-
triathlete-michael-giardino-died-doing-what-he-loved (48
yr old male)

https://www.timeslive.co.za/news/south-
africa/2013-01-22-ironman-fatality-was-out-to-win/ (28
yr old male and 36 yr old male)

https://www.cnn.com/2013/03/03/us/california-triathlon-death/index.html (46 yr old male)

2012:

http://boston.cbslocal.com/2012/08/19/beverly-man-dies-in-vermont-triathlon/ (53 yr old male)

https://www.nytimes.com/2012/08/12/nyregion/man-dies-during-swim-leg-of-ironman-triathlon.html (43 yr old male)

http://www.spokesman.com/stories/2012/jun/27/seattle-man-dies-after-coeur-dalene-ironman-swim/ (44 yr old male)

http://fox6now.com/2012/06/17/illinois-man-drowns-in-wisconsin-triathlon/ (42 yr old male)

https://www.wsbtv.com/news/widow-wants-answers-husbands-triathlon-death/242399019 (43 yr old male)

2011:

http://www.triathlete.com/2011/08/news/second-participant-in-new-york-city-triathlon-dies_36257 (40 yr old woman, 64 yr old man)

https://www.medicalnewstoday.com/articles/226851.php (42 yr old male)

http://www.wdrb.com/story/15348474/athlete-dies-at-the-ironman (46 yr old male)

2010:

http://abcnews.go.com/Health/Wellness/fran-crippen-death-heat-stroke-heart-problems/story?id=11967179 (26 yr old male)

2009:

https://www.twincities.com/2009/08/09/woman-43-dies-during-oshkosh-triathlon/ (43 yr old woman)

http://www.asiaone.com/News/AsiaOne%2BNews/Singapore/Story/A1Story20090803-158676.html (42 yr old male)

http://www.nbc15.com/home/headlines/53349887.html (38 yr old woman)

http://www.cbc.ca/news/canada/british-columbia/alberta-senior-dies-during-b-c-ironman-swim-1.779872 (66 yr old male)

http://archive.jsonline.com/news/obituaries/48117632.html/ (54 yr old woman)

https://www.twincities.com/2009/07/13/man-who-died-in-wisconsin-triathlon-had-lost-100-pounds-in-training/ (33 yr old male)

2008:

https://www.nytimes.com/2008/07/21/sports/othersports/21triathlon.html (32 yr old male)

https://www.sfgate.com/bayarea/article/Swimmer-63-dies-during-Alcatraz-triathlon-3198607.php (63 yr old male)

https://www.idahopress.com/news/utahn-dies-during-spudman-triathlon-in-burley/article_ad8f439e-2750-5e5a-8574-2317a1780b72.html (60 yr old male)

https://www.chron.com/news/houston-texas/article/Conroe-man-who-died-in-triathlon-had-years-of-1783052.php (51 year old male)

http://www.nj.com/news/index.ssf/2008/07/triath
letes_body_found_in_lake.html (52 yr old male)

2007:
http://articles.orlandosentinel.com/2009-10-
12/news/0910100053_1_triathlon-anoxic-
encephalopathy-santa-maria (43 yr old woman)
http://www.stltoday.com/suburban-
journals/athlete-dies-during-ultramax-
triathlon/article_8cd5ded7-c582-548b-9aab-
7fbf671d80f7.html (28 yr old male)

2005:
https://www.denverpost.com/2005/07/26/particip
ant-dies-another-hurt-in-boulder-triathlon/ (76 yr old
male)
http://www.sgrunners.com/forum/index.php?/cale
ndar/event/67-ho-wai-piew-memorial-run/ (40 yr old
male)

2002:
http://www.grandrapidsmn.com/news/illinois-man-
dies-while-competing-in-timberman-
triathlon/article_cf433575-9e48-50af-a0b5-
63fd5035330f.html (36 yr old male)

1995:
http://articles.chicagotribune.com/1995-08-
29/news/9508290121_1_triathlon-federation-triathlon-
competition-heart-disease (39 yr old male)

Studies on Marathon Death Rates

Competing risks of mortality with marathons: retrospective analysis. Donald A Redelmeier, and J Ari Greenwald, BMJ. 2007 Dec 22; 335(7633): 1275–1277. doi: 10.1136/bmj.39384.551539.25

https://www.ncbi.nlm.nih.gov/pmc/articles/PMC2151171/

Risk for sudden cardiac death associated with marathon running.

Maron BJ, Poliac LC, Roberts WO. J Am Coll Cardiol. 1996 Aug 28(2): 428-31.

http://www.ncbi.nlm.nih.gov/pubmed/8800121

London Marathon: incidence of injury, illness and death. Andrew Hamilton. Endurance Health and Lifestyle. http://www.pponline.co.uk/encyc/london-marathon-what-we-know-about-the-incidence-of-injury-illness-and-death-in-the-london-marathon-881#

Scientific Papers on Physiological Aspects of Open Water Swimming

(a) I. Warming-up for Swimming

1. **Does warm-up have a beneficial effect on 100-m freestyle?** Neiva HP, Marques MC, Fernandes RJ, Viana JL, Barbosa TM, Marinho DA. Int J Sports Physiol Perform. 2014 Jan; 9(1): 145-50.PMID: 23579194.

2. **Warm-up and performance in competitive swimming**. Neiva HP, Marques MC, Barbosa TM, Izquierdo M, Marinho DA. Sports Med. 2014 Mar; 44(3): 319-30.PMID: 24178508.

3. **Effects of different types of warm-up on swimming performance, reaction time, and dive distance**. Balilionis G, Nepocatych S, Ellis CM, Richardson MT, Neggers YH, Bishop PA. J Strength Cond Res. 2012 Dec; 26(12): 3297-303. PMID: 22237141.

4. **Effect of different warm-up procedures on subsequent swim and overall sprint distance triathlon performance**. Binnie MJ, Landers G, Peeling P. J Strength Cond Res. 2012 Sep 26(9): 2438-46. PMID: 22067241.

5. **The Effect of Warm-up on Tethered Front Crawl Swimming Forces**. Neiva H, Morouço P, Silva AJ, Marques MC, Marinho DA. Journal of Human Kinetics. 2011:113-9.PMID: SportDiscus: 70838706.

6. **Stretching and injury prevention: An enigmatic relationship [Conference Abstract]**. Witvrouw E, Ahieu N, McNair P. Journal of Science and Medicine in Sport. 2011 December 14: e95-e6. PMID: EMBASE: 70686060.

7. **Effects of prolonged and reduced warm-ups on diurnal variation in body temperature and swim performance**. Arnett MG. J Strength Cond Res. 2002 May; 16(2): 256-61.PMID: 11991779.

8. **The effect of high- and low-intensity warm-up on the physiological responses to a standardized swim and tethered swimming performance**. Mitchell JB, Huston JS. J Sports Sci. 1993 Apr; 11(2): 159-65.PMID: 8497018.

9. **The effect of warm-up on responses to intense exercise**. Houmard JA, Johns RA, Smith LL, Wells JM, Kobe RW, McGoogan SA. Int J Sports Med. 1991 Oct; 12(5): 480-3.PMID:

(b) II. Sleep Deprivation and Sleep Performance

1. **The body clock and athletic performance [Conference Abstract]**. Reilly T. Biological Rhythm Research. 2009 February 40(1): 37-44. EMBASE: 2008597280.

2. **Circadian variation in swim performance**. Kline CE, Durstine JL, Davis JM, Moore TA, Devlin TM, Zielinski MR, Youngstedt SD. Journal of Applied Physiology. 2007; 102(2): 641-9. SportDiscus:

24101953.

3. **An evaluation of pre-participation self-assessment for triathlon and aquathon**. Kasanami R, Tanaka Y, Umegaki Y, Kiyonari N, Takakura Y, Kurumatani N. Japanese Journal of Clinical Sports Medicine. 2006; 14(3): 316-24. SportDiscus: 23832203.

4. **Sleep deprivation and the effect on exercise performance**. VanHelder T, Radomski MW. Sports Med. 1989 Apr; 7(4): 235-47.PMID: 2657963.

(c) III. Drowning Mechanisms

1. **Near drowning and adult respiratory distress syndrome**. Buggia M, Canham L, Tibbles C, Landry A. J Emerg Med. 2014 Jun; 46(6): 821-5. PMID: 24642043.

2. **Habituation of the Cold Shock Response May Include a Significant Perceptual Component**. Barwood MJ, Corbett JO, Wagstaff CRD. Aerospace Medicine & Human Performance. 2014; 85(2): 167-71. SportDiscus: 94065067.

3. **Airway obstruction due to aspiration of muddy water**. Schober P, Christiaans HMT, Loer SA, Schwarte LA. Emergency Medicine Journal. 2013 October; 30(10): 854-5. EMBASE: 2013601775.

4. **Post-mortem visceral water contents in drowning: A pilot study**. Kawamoto O, Ishikawa T, Michiue T, Maeda H. Rechtsmedizin. 2012 August; 22 (4): 351. EMBASE: 71620784.

5. **Failure to ventilate with supraglottic airways after drowning**. Baker PA, Webber JB. Anaesth

Intensive Care. 2011 Jul; 39(4): 675-7. PMID: 21823389.

6. **Two cases of drowning and "delayed death from drowning" while the victims scuba-dived together**. Kubo H, Hayashi T, Ago K, Ago M, Nakashima H, Ogata M. Rechtsmedizin. 2011 August; 21 (4): 411. EMBASE.

7. **Pulmonary molecular pathology of drowning**. Miyazato T, Ishikawa T, Michiue T, Maeda H.Rechtsmedizin. 2010 August; 20 (4): 345. EMBASE: 71620834.

8. **Near-drowning and clinical laboratory changes**. Oehmichen M, Hennig R, Meissner C. Legal Medicine. 2008 January; 10(1): 1-5. EMBASE: 2007575033.

9. **Salt water aspiration syndrome**. Mitchell S. South Pacific Underwater Medicine Society Journal. 2002 December; 32(4): 205-6. EMBASE: 2003014107.

10. **The pathophysiology of drowning**. North R. South Pacific Underwater Medicine Society Journal. 2002 December 32(4): 194-7. EMBASE: 2003014104.

11. **Drowning. Rescue, resuscitation, and reanimation**. Orlowski JP, Szpilman D. Pediatr Clin North Am. 2001 Jun; 48(3): 627-46.PMID: 11411297.

12. **Drowning syndromes: the mechanism**. Edmonds C. SPUMS Journal. 1998; 28(1): 2-9. SportDiscus: SPH463111.

13. **A case of deferred death from drowning of a man found dead in bed at home**. Sato Y, Kondo T, Ohshima T. Journal of Clinical Forensic Medicine. 1996; 3(2): 105-7. EMBASE: 1996307698.

14. **Near-drowning**. Bross MH, Clark JL. Am Fam Physician. 1995 May 1; 51(6): 1545-51, 55. PMID: 7732954.

15. **Drowning issues in resuscitation**. Quan L. Ann Emerg Med. 1993 Feb; 22(Pt 2): 366-9.PMID: 8434835.

16. **Why some people do not drown. Hypothermia versus the diving response**. Gooden BA. Med J Aust. 1992 Nov 2; 157(9): 629-32.PMID: 1406426.

17. **Near-drowning: fresh, salt, and cold water immersion**. Sarnaik AP, Vohra MP. Clinics in Sports Medicine. 1986; 5(1): 33-46. SportDiscus: SPH179755.

18. **Swimming and loss of consciousness**. Suzuki T, Ikeda N, Umetsu K, Kashimura S. Z Rechtsmed. 1985; 94(2): 121-6.PMID: 4002881.

19. **A salt water aspiration syndrome**. Edmonds C. Mil Med. 1970 Sep; 135(9): 779-85.PMID: 4991232.

20. **Resuscitation following fresh-water or sea-water aspiration**. Safar P. Acta Anaesthesiol Scand Suppl. 1961;Suppl 9:99-108.PMID: 14495973.

21. **How much did cold shock and swimming failure contribute to drowning deaths in the fishing industry in British Columbia 1976-2002?** Brooks CJ[1], Howard KA, Neifer SK. Occup Med (Lond). 2005 Sep; 55(6): 459-62. Epub 2005 May 4.

22. **Clinical, laboratory and X-ray findings of drowning and near-drowning in the Gulf of Aqaba.** al-Talafieh A, al-Majali R, al-Dehayat G. East Mediterr

Health J. 1999 Jul; 5(4): 706-9.PMID: 11338693.

23. **Drowning and near-drowning — some lessons learnt**. Goh SH, Low BY. Ann Acad Med Singapore. 1999 Mar; 28(2): 183-8.PMID: 10497663.

24. **'Autonomic conflict': a different way to die during cold water immersion?** Michael J Shattock and Michael J Tipton. J Physiol. 2012 Jul 15; 590(Pt 14): 3219–3230.

Published online 2012 Apr 30. doi: 10.1113/jphysiol.2012.229864 PMCID: PMC3459038

PMID: 22547634

25. **Physiology Of Drowning: A Review.** Joost J. L. M. Bierens, Philippe Lunetta, Mike Tipton, and David S. Warner. 17 FEB 2016 https://doi.org/10.1152/physiol.00002.2015

(d) IV. The Effects of Cold Water Immersion

1. **Idiopathic cold urticaria and anaphylaxis**. Isk S, Arkan-Ayyldz Z, Sozmen SC, Karaman O, Uzuner N. Pediatr Emerg Care. 2014 Jan; 30(1): 38-9. PMID: 24378859.

2. **Responses to sudden cold-water immersion in inexperienced swimmers following training**. Croft JL, Button C, Hodge K, Lucas SJ, Barwood MJ, Cotter JD. Aviat Space Environ Med. 2013 Aug; 84(8): 850-5.PMID: 23926662.

3. **Effect of winter swimming on haematological parameters**. Lombardi G, Ricci C, Banfi G. Biochem

Med (Zagreb). 2011; 21(1): 71-8. PMID: 22141210.

4. **Hypothermia in open-water swimming events: a medical risk that deserves more attention**. de Castro RR, da Nobrega AC. Wilderness Environ Med. 2009 Winter; 20(4): 394-5; author reply 5. PMID: 20030455.

5. **Hypothermia is a significant medical risk of mass participation long-distance open water swimming**. Brannigan D, Rogers IR, Jacobs I, Montgomery A, Williams A, Khangure N. Wilderness Environ Med. 2009 Spring; 20(1): 14-8. PMID: 19364182.

6. **Cold-induced anaphylaxis**. Fernando SL. J Pediatr. 2009 Jan; 154(1): 148- e1. PMID: 19187742.

7. **Asthma, airway inflammation and epithelial damage in swimmers and cold-air athletes**. Bougault V, Turmel J, St-Laurent J, Bertrand M, Boulet LP. Eur Respir J. 2009 Apr; 33(4): 740-6. PMID: 19129276.

8. **Swimming in ice cold water**. Knechtle B, Christinger N, Kohler G, Knechtle P, Rosemann T. Ir J Med Sci. 2009 Dec; 178(4): 507-11.PMID: 19763672.

9. **Arm insulation and swimming in cold water**. Lounsbury DS, Ducharme MB. Eur J Appl Physiol. 2008 Sep; 104(2): 159-74. PMID: 18309510.

10. **Modulation of adrenergic receptors and adrenergic functions in cold adapted humans**. Jansky L, Vybiral S, Trubacova M, Okrouhlik J. Eur J Appl Physiol. 2008 Sep; 104(2): 131-5. PMID: 18060558.

11. **Self-rescue swimming in cold water: the latest advice**. Ducharme MB, Lounsbury DS. Appl Physiol Nutr Metab. 2007 Aug; 32(4): 799-807.PMID: 17622298.

12. **Thermal insulation and body temperature wearing a thermal swimsuit during water immersion**. Wakabayashi H, Hanai A, Yokoyama S, Nomura T. J Physiol Anthropol. 2006 Sep; 25(5): 331-8. PMID: 17016009.

13. **How much did cold shock and swimming failure contribute to drowning deaths in the fishing industry in British Columbia 1976-2002?** Brooks CJ, Howard KA, Neifer SK. Occup Med (Lond). 2005 Sep; 55(6): 459-62. PMID: 15871996.

14. **Thermal sensation and comfort in women exposed repeatedly to whole-body cryotherapy and winter swimming in ice-cold water**. Smolander J, Mikkelsson M, Oksa J, Westerlund T, Leppaluoto J, Huttunen P. Physiol Behav. 2004 Sep 30; 82(4): 691-5. PMID: 15327918.

15. **The physiology of channel swimmers. 1955**. Pugh LG, Edholm OG. Wilderness Environ Med. 2004 Spring; 15(1): 40-1; discussion 38-9. PMID: 15043005.

16. **Winter swimming: healthy or hazardous? Evidence and hypotheses**. Kolettis TM, Kolettis MT. Med Hypotheses. 2003 Nov-Dec; 61(5-6): 654-6. PMID: 14592803.

17. **Neurotic psychopathology and alexithymia among winter swimmers and controls — a prospective study**. Lindeman S, Hirvonen J, Joukamaa M. Int J Circumpolar Health. 2002 May; 61(2): 123-30.PMID: 12078959.

18. **Effect of regular winter swimming on the activity of the sympathoadrenal system before and**

after a single cold water immersion. Huttunen P, Rintamaki H, Hirvonen J. Int J Circumpolar Health. 2001 Aug; 60(3): 400-6.PMID: 11590880.

19. **Exercise and the cold**. Noakes TD. Ergonomics. 2000 Oct; 43(10): 1461-79. PMID: 11083128.

20. **Adaptation related to cytokines in man: effects of regular swimming in ice-cold water**. Dugue B, Leppanen E. Clin Physiol. 2000 Mar; 20(2): 114-21. PMID: 10735978.

21. **Thermography in front crawl swimming at anaerobic threshold intensity [Conference Abstract]**. Dejesus K, Ramos A, Vilas Boas JP, Gabriel J. Thermology International. 2012 July; 22 (3): 107-8. EMBASE: 70892446.

22. **Effect of non-uniform skin temperature on thermoregulatory response during water immersion**. Wakabayashi H, Kaneda K, Sato D, Tochihara Y, Nomura T. Eur J Appl Physiol. 2008 Sep; 104(2): 175-81. PMID: 18351380.

23. **The Mammalian Diving Response: An Enigmatic Reflex to Preserve Life?** W. Michael Panneton. Physiology (Bethesda). 2013 Sep; 28(5): 284–297. doi: 10.1152/physiol.00020.2013 PMCID: PMC3768097 PMID: 23997188

(e) V. Respiratory Compromise: General

1. Integrative physiological and behavioural responses to sudden cold-water immersion are

similar in skilled and less-skilled swimmers. Button C, Croft JL, Cotter JD, Graham MJ, Lucas SJE. Physiology and Behaviour. 2015 January 01; 138:254-9. EMBASE: <u>2014929834</u>.

2. **Breathing manoeuvre-dependent changes in myocardial oxygenation in healthy humans**. Guensch DP, Fischer K, Flewitt JA, Yu J, Lukic R, Friedrich JA, Friedrich MG. Eur Heart J Cardiovasc Imaging. 2014 Apr; 15(4): 409-14.PMID: 24078154.

3. **Don't hold your breath: Anoxic convulsions from coupled hyperventilation-underwater breath-holding**. Kumar KR, Ng K. Medical Journal of Australia. 2010 07 Jun; 192(11): 663-4.

4. **Scientific Review: Avoiding Hyperventilation**. International Journal of Aquatic Research & Education. 2009; 3(4): 432-47. SportDiscus: 45306142.

5. **Aggravated hypoxia during breath-holds after prolonged exercise**. Lindholm P, Gennser M. European Journal of Applied Physiology. 2005 March; 93(5-6): 701-7. EMBASE: 2005146033.

6. **Airway cells after swimming outdoors or in the sea in nonasthmatic athletes**. Bonsignore MR, Morici G, Riccobono L, Profita M, Bonanno A, Paterno A, Di Giorgi R, Chimenti L, Abate P, Mirabella F, et al. Medicine and Science in Sports and Exercise. 2003 01 Jul; 35(7): 1146-52. EMBASE: 2003273506.

7. **Exertional dizziness and autonomic dysregulation**. Staab JP, Ruckenstein MJ, Solomon D, Shepard NT. Laryngoscope. 2002; 112(8 I): 1346-50. EMBASE: 2002287263.

8. **Voluntary hyperventilation as a cause of needless drowning**. Snively WD, Jr., Thuerbach J. R I Med J. 1972 Jun; 55(6): 193-6 passim. PMID: 4504749.

9. **Sudden failure of swimming in cold water**. Keatinge WR, Prys-Roberts C, Cooper KE, Honour AJ, Haight J. Br Med J. 1969 Feb 22; 1(5642): 480-3. PMID: 5764250.

10. **Death in cold water**. Med J Aust. 1969 Mar 29; 1(13): 693. PMID: 5769461.

11. **Physiological aspects of mammalian breath-hold diving: a review**. Strauss MB. Aerosp Med. 1970 Dec; 41(12): 1362-81.PMID: 4922840.

12. **Exercise induced arterial hypoxemia in swimmers**. Spanoudaki SS, Maridaki MD, Myrianthefs PM, Baltopoulos PJ. J Sports Med & Phys Fitness. 2004; 44(4): 342-8. SportDiscus: SPHS-997735.

13. **The comparison of peak oxygen uptake between swim-bench exercise and arm stroke**. Ogita F, Taniguchi S. Eur J Appl Physiol Occup Physiol. 1995; 71(4): 295-300.PMID: 8549570.

(f) VI. Respiratory Compromise: Swimming Induced Pulmonary Edema (SIPE)

1. **Swimming-induced pulmonary oedema in two triathletes: a novel pathophysiological explanation**. Casey H, Dastidar AG, MacIver D. J R Soc Med. 2014 Nov; 107(11): 450-2. PMID: 25341446.

2. **Extreme sports: extreme physiology. Exercise-induced pulmonary oedema**. Ma JL, Dutch

MJ. Emerg Med Australas. 2013 Aug; 25(4): 368-71. PMID: 23911030.

3. **Swimming-induced immersion pulmonary edema while snorkelling can be rapidly life-threatening: case reports**. Cochard G, Henckes A, Deslandes S, Noel-Savina E, Bedossa M, Gladu G, Ozier Y. Undersea Hyperb Med. 2013 Sep-Oct; 40(5): 411-6.PMID: 24224285.

4. **A case of acute breathlessness in a swimmer**. North VJ, Mansfield H. Emerg Med J. 2013 May; 30(5): 429. PMID: 23175704.

5. **Early subclinical increase in pulmonary water content in athletes performing sustained heavy exercise at sea level: ultrasound lung comet-tail evidence**. Pingitore A, Garbella E, Piaggi P, Menicucci D, Frassi F, Lionetti V, Piarulli A, Catapano G, Lubrano V, Passera M, et al. Am J Physiol Heart Circ Physiol. 2011 Nov; 301(5): H2161-7. PMID: 21873499.

6. **Swimming-induced pulmonary edema in triathletes**. Miller CC, 3rd, Calder-Becker K, Modave F. Am J Emerg Med. 2010 Oct; 28(8): 941-6. PMID: 20887912.

7. **Effects of hyperoxia on ventilation and pulmonary hemodynamics during immersed prone exercise at 4.7 ATA: possible implications for immersion pulmonary edema**. Peacher DF, Pecorella SR, Freiberger JJ, Natoli MJ, Schinazi EA, Doar PO, Boso AE, Walker AJ, Gill M, Kernagis D, et al. J Appl Physiol (1985). 2010 Jul; 109(1): 68-78. PMID: 20431020.

8. **Swimming-induced pulmonary oedema — a**

hazard in intensive military training? Knutson T. J R Army Med Corps. 2010 Dec; 156(4): 258-9.PMID: 21275362.

9. **Brain natriuretic peptide levels in six basic underwater demolitions/SEAL recruits presenting with swimming induced pulmonary edema (SIPE).** Shearer D, Mahon R. J Spec Oper Med. 2009 Summer; 9(3): 44-50. PMID: 19739476.

10. **Novel presentation of acute pericarditis in an Ironman triathlete.** Pearce PZ. Curr Sports Med Rep. 2007 Jun; 6(3): 179-82. PMID: 19202664.

11. **Cold water-induced pulmonary edema.** Beinart R, Matetzky S, Arad T, Hod H. Am J Med. 2007 Sep; 120(9): e3. PMID: 17765034.

12. **Scuba diving, swimming and pulmonary oedema.** Dwyer N, Smart D, Reid DW. Intern Med J. 2007 May; 37(5): 345-7. PMID: 17504290.

13. **Cardiopulmonary function after recovery from swimming-induced pulmonary edema.** Ludwig BB, Mahon RT, Schwartzman EL. Clin J Sport Med. 2006 Jul; 16(4): 348-51. PMID: 16858220.

14. **A swimmer's wheeze.** Deady B, Glezo J, Blackie S. CJEM. 2006 Jul;8(4): 281, 97-8.PMID: 17324310.

15. **Acute pulmonary edema during a triathlon occurrence in a trained athlete.** Boggio-Alarco JL, Jaume-Anselmi F, Ramirez-Rivera J. Bol Assoc Med P R. 2006 Apr-Jun; 98(2): 110-3.PMID: 19606798.

16. **Pulmonary oedema of immersion.** Koehle MS, Lepawsky M, McKenzie DC. Sports Med. 2005; 35(3):

183-90.PMID: 15730335.

17. **Pulmonary oedema precipitated by cold water swimming**. Biswas R, Shibu PK, James CM. Br J Sports Med. 2004 Dec; 38(6): e36. PMID: 15562151.

18. **Management of swimming-induced pulmonary edema**. Yoder JA, Viera AJ. Am Fam Physician. 2004 Mar 1; 69(5): 1046, 8-9. PMID: 15023003.

19. **Swimming-induced pulmonary edema: clinical presentation and serial lung function**. Adir Y, Shupak A, Gil A, Peled N, Keynan Y, Domachevsky L, Weiler-Ravell D. Chest. 2004 Aug;126(2):394-9.PMID: 15302723.

20. **Swimming-induced pulmonary edema**. Lund KL, Mahon RT, Tanen DA, Bakhda S. Ann Emerg Med. 2003 Feb;41(2):251-6. PMID: 12548277.

21. **Immersion pulmonary edema in Special Forces combat swimmers**. Mahon RT, Kerr S, Amundson D, Parrish JS. Chest. 2002 Jul;122(1):383-4.PMID: 12114391.

22. **Pulmonary oedema induced by strenuous swimming: a field study**. Shupak A, Weiler-Ravell D, Adir Y, Daskalovic YI, Ramon Y, Kerem D. Respir Physiol. 2000 Jun; 121(1): 25-31.PMID: 10854620.

23. **Pulmonary oedema in healthy persons during scuba-diving and swimming**. Pons M, Blickenstorfer D, Oechslin E, Hold G, Greminger P, Franzeck UK, Russi EW. Eur Respir J. 1995 May; 8(5): 762-7. PMID: 7656948.

24. **Pulmonary oedema and hemoptysis induced**

by strenuous swimming.

Weiler-Ravell D, Shupak A, Goldenberg I, Halpern P, Shoshani O, Hirschhorn G, Margulis A. BMJ. 1995 Aug 5; 311(7001): 361-2. PMID: 7640542.

25. **Cold-induced pulmonary oedema in scuba divers and swimmers and subsequent development of hypertension**. Wilmshurst PT, Nuri M, Crowther A, Webb-Peploe MM. Lancet. 1989 Jan 14; 1(8629): 62-5.PMID: 2562880.

26. **SIPE: A price for a prize [Conference Abstract]**. Chandra M, Nuckton TJ. Journal of General Internal Medicine. 2015 April; 30:S318. EMBASE: 71878048.

27. **A triathlete with acute onset of dyspnea and hemoptysis [Conference Abstract]**. Pintscher K, Hubner M, Kneussl M. European Respiratory Journal. 2014 01 Sep; 44. EMBASE: 71849906.

28. **Moving in extreme environments: Open water swimming in cold and warm water**. Tipton M, Bradford C. Extreme Physiology and Medicine. 2014 11 Jun; 3(1). EMBASE: 2014399189.

29. **A case of recurrent swimming-induced pulmonary edema in a triathlete: the need for awareness**. Smith R, Brooke D, Kipps C, Skaria B, Subramaniam V. Scand J Med Sci Sports. 2017 Oct; 27(10): 1130-1135. doi: 10.1111/sms. 12736. Epub 2016 Aug 3.

(g) VII. Gastrointestinal Issues: Effects of

Food, Supplements and Water

1. **Nutrition considerations for open-water swimming**. Shaw G, Koivisto A, Gerrard D, Burke LM. Int J Sport Nutr Exerc Metab. 2014 Aug; 24(4): 373-81.PMID: 24667305.

2. **Nutritional intake and gastrointestinal problems during competitive endurance events**. Pfeiffer B, Stellingwerff T, Hodgson AB, Randell R, Pottgen K, Res P, Jeukendrup AE. Med Sci Sports Exerc. 2012 Feb; 44(2): 344-51. PMID: 21775906.

3. **Body composition and hydration status changes in male and female open-water swimmers during an ultra-endurance event**. Weitkunat T, Knechtle B, Knechtle P, Rust CA, Rosemann T. J Sports Sci. 2012; 30(10): 1003-13.PMID: 22554315.

4. **Increased running speed and previous cramps rather than dehydration or serum sodium changes predict exercise-associated muscle cramping: a prospective cohort study in 210 Ironman triathletes**. Schwellnus MP, Drew N, Collins M. Br J Sports Med. 2011 Jun; 45(8): 650-6. PMID: 21148567.

5. **Survey results of the training, nutrition, and mental preparation of triathletes: practical implications of findings**. Dolan SH, Houston M, Martin SB. J Sports Sci. 2011 Jul; 29(10): 1019-28. PMID: 21623532.

6. **Race-day carbohydrate intakes of elite triathletes contesting olympic-distance triathlon events**. Cox GR, Snow RJ, Burke LM. Int J Sport Nutr Exerc Metab. 2010 Aug; 20(4): 299-306.PMID:

20739718.

7. **Water and salt balance of well-trained swimmers in training**. Maughan RJ, Dargavel LA, Hares R, Shirreffs SM. Int J Sport Nutr Exerc Metab. 2009 Dec; 19(6): 598-606. PMID: 20175429.

8. **Hyperthermic fatigue precedes a rapid reduction in serum sodium in an ironman triathlete: a case report**. Laursen PB, Watson G, Abbiss CR, Wall BA, Nosaka K. Int J Sports Physiol Perform. 2009 Dec; 4(4): 533-7. PMID: 20029104.

9. **Antihistamine and sodium cromoglycate medication for food cold water exercise-induced anaphylaxis**. Benhamou AH, Vanini G, Lantin JP, Eigenmann PA. Allergy. 2007 Dec; 62(12): 1471-2. PMID: 17983384.

10. **Moderate exercise-induced hyponatremia**. Shapiro SA, Ejaz AA, Osborne MD, Taylor WC. Clin J Sport Med. 2006 Jan; 16(1): 72-3. PMID: 16377980.

11. **The timing of fluid intake during an Olympic distance triathlon**. McMurray RG, Williams DK, Battaglini CL. Int J Sport Nutr Exerc Metab. 2006 Dec; 16(6): 611-9.PMID: 17342882.

12. **Comparison of water turnover rates in young swimmers in training and age-matched non-training individuals**. Leiper JB, Maughan RJ. Int J Sport Nutr Exerc Metab. 2004 Jun; 14(3): 347-57. PMID: 15256694.

13. **Dietary intake and energy expenditure of female collegiate swimmers during decreased training prior to competition**. Ousley-Pahnke L, Black DR, Gretebeck RJ. J Am Diet Assoc. 2001 Mar; 101(3):

351-4. PMID: 11269618.

14. **Effect of overhydration on time-trial swim performance**. Maresh CM, Bergeron MF, Kenefick RW, Castellani JW, Hoffman JR, Armstrong LE. J Strength Cond Res. 2001 Nov; 15(4): 514-8.PMID: 11726266.

15. **The effects of aerobic and anaerobic exercise conditioning on resting metabolic rate and the thermic effect of a meal**. Schmidt WD, Hyner GC, Lyle RM, Corrigan D, Bottoms G, Melby CL. Int J Sport Nutr. 1994 Dec; 4(4): 335-46. PMID: 7874150.

16. **Dietary intervention and training in swimmers**. Cade JR, Reese RH, Privette RM, Hommen NM, Rogers JL, Fregly MJ. Eur J Appl Physiol Occup Physiol. 1991; 63(3-4): 210-5.PMID: 1761010.

17. **Eating and training habits of triathletes: a balancing act**. Lindeman AK. J Am Diet Assoc. 1990 Jul; 90(7): 993-5. PMID: 2365944.

18. **Sodium bicarbonate ingestion improves performance in interval swimming**. Gao JP, Costill DL, Horswill CA, Park SH. Eur J Appl Physiol Occup Physiol. 1988; 58(1-2): 171-4. PMID: 2849539.

19. **Nutrition for swimmers**. Grandjean AC. Clin Sports Med. 1986 Jan; 5(1): 65-76. PMID: 3512105.

20. **Effect of food consumption on 200-yard freestyle swim performance**. Singer RN, Neeves RE. Res Q. 1968 May; 39(2): 355-60. PMID: 5240118.

21. **Effect of eating at various times on subsequent performances in the one-mile freestyle swim**. Asprey GM, Alley LE, Tuttle WW. Res Q. 1968 May; 39(2): 231-4. PMID: 5240100.

22. **Dietary supplements for aquatic sports**.
Derave W, Tipton KD. Int J Sport Nutr Exerc Metab.
2014 Aug; 24(4): 437-49. PMID: 24667103.

(h) VIII. Food Substrates on Performance

1. **Meal induced gut hormone secretion is altered in aerobically trained compared to sedentary young healthy males**. Lund MT, Taudorf L, Hartmann B, Helge JW, Holst JJ, Dela F. Eur J Appl Physiol. 2013 Nov; 113(11): 2737-47. PMID: 23979179.

2. **Dietary protein digestion and absorption are impaired during acute post-exercise recovery in young men**. van Wijck K, Pennings B, van Bijnen AA, Senden JM, Buurman WA, Dejong CH, van Loon LJ, Lenaerts K. Am J Physiol Regul Integr Comp Physiol. 2013 Mar 1; 304(5): R356-61. PMID: 23283940.

3. **Metabolism and performance during extended high-intensity intermittent exercise after consumption of low- and high-glycemic index pre-exercise meals**. Bennett CB, Chilibeck PD, Barss T, Vatanparast H, Vandenberg A, Zello GA. Br J Nutr. 2012 Aug; 108 Suppl 1: S81-90. PMID: 22916819.

4. **Effect of glycemic index meals on recovery and subsequent endurance capacity**. Wong SH, Chen YJ, Fung WM, Morris JG. Int J Sports Med. 2009 Dec; 30(12): 898-905. PMID: 20013559.

5. **The effect of acute exercise on endothelial function following a high-fat meal**. Padilla J, Harris RA, Fly AD, Rink LD, Wallace JP. Eur J Appl Physiol.

2006 Oct; 98(3): 256-62. PMID: 16896723.

6. **Metabolic responses to exercise after carbohydrate loads in healthy men and women**. Leelayuwat N, Tsintzas K, Patel K, Macdonald IA. Med Sci Sports Exerc. 2005 Oct; 37(10): 1721-7. PMID: 16260972.

7. **The influence of the glycaemic index of breakfast and lunch on substrate utilisation during the postprandial periods and subsequent exercise**. Stevenson E, Williams C, Nute M. Br J Nutr. 2005 Jun; 93(6): 885-93. PMID: 16022758.

8. **Effect of frequency of carbohydrate feedings on recovery and subsequent endurance run**. Siu PM, Wong SH, Morris JG, Lam CW, Chung PK, Chung S. Med Sci Sports Exerc. 2004 Feb; 36(2): 315-23. PMID: 14767257.

9. **The influence of high-carbohydrate meals with different glycaemic indices on substrate utilisation during subsequent exercise**. Wu CL, Nicholas C, Williams C, Took A, Hardy L. Br J Nutr. 2003 Dec; 90(6): 1049-56. PMID: 14641964.

10. **Lower oxidation of a high molecular weight glucose polymer vs. glucose during cycling**. Rowlands DS, Clarke J. Applied Physiology, Nutrition & Metabolism. 2011; 36(2): 298-306. SportDiscus: 65516255.

(i) IX. Digestive Processes and Swimming

1. **Duodenal motility during a run-bike-run**

protocol: the effect of a sports drink. Peters HP, de Vries WR, Akkermans LM, van Berge-Henegouwen GP, Koerselman J, Wiersma JW, Bol E, Mosterd WL. Eur J Gastroenterol Hepatol. 2002 Oct; 14(10): 1125-32. PMID: 12362104.

2. **Gastrointestinal problems as a function of carbohydrate supplements and mode of exercise.** Peters HP, Van Schelven FW, Verstappen PA, De Boer RW, Bol E, Erich WB, Van Der Togt CR, De Vries W. Medicine & Science in Sports & Exercise. 1993; 25(11): 1211-24. SportDiscus: SPH343313.

3. **Gastrointestinal symptoms during exercise in Enduro athletes: prevalence and speculations on the aetiology.** Worobetz LJ, Gerrard DF. N Z Med J. 1985 Aug 14; 98(784): 644-6. PMID: 3861978.

(j) X. Digestive Processes and Exercise Generally

1. **Acute Exercise and Gastric Emptying: A Meta-Analysis and Implications for Appetite Control.** Horner K, Schubert M, Desbrow B, Byrne N, King N. Sports Medicine. 2015; 45(5): 659-78. SportDiscus: 102202418.

2. **Gastrointestinal Complaints During Exercise: Prevalence, Etiology, and Nutritional Recommendations.** Oliveira E, Burini R, Jeukendrup A. Sports Medicine. 2014; 44: 79-85. SportDiscus: 95865972.

3. **Water intake accelerates parasympathetic reactivation after high-intensity exercise.** Pecanha T,

Paula-Ribeiro M, Campana-Rezende E, Bartels R, Marins JC, de Lima JR. Int J Sport Nutr Exerc Metab. 2014 Oct; 24(5): 489-96. PMID: 24667231.

4. **Review article: the pathophysiology and management of gastrointestinal symptoms during physical exercise, and the role of splanchnic blood flow.** ter Steege RW, Kolkman JJ. Aliment Pharmacol Ther. 2012 Mar; 35(5): 516-28. PMID: 22229513.

5. **Influence of endurance training on central sympathetic outflow to skeletal muscle in response to a mixed meal.** Young CN, Deo SH, Kim A, Horiuchi M, Mikus CR, Uptergrove GM, Thyfault JP, Fadel PJ. J Appl Physiol (1985). 2010 Apr; 108(4): 882-90. PMID: 20110544.

6. **Water intake accelerates post-exercise cardiac vagal reactivation in humans.** Vianna LC, Oliveira RB, Silva BM, Ricardo DR, Araujo CG. Eur J Appl Physiol. 2008 Feb; 102(3): 283-8. PMID: 17929050.

7. **The effects of physical activity on the gastrointestinal tract.** Strid H, Simrén M. International SportMed Journal. 2005; 6(3): 151-61. SportDiscus: 26316916.

8. **Effect of intermittent high-intensity exercise on gastric emptying in man.** Leiper JB, Broad NP, Maughan RJ. Medicine & Science in Sports & Exercise. 2001; 33(8): 1270-8. SportDiscus: SPHS-786579.

9. **Intestinal fluid absorption during exercise: role of sport drink osmolality and (Na+).** Gisolfi CV, Lambert GP, Summers RW. Medicine & Science in Sports & Exercise. 2001; 33(6): 907-15. SportDiscus:

SPHS-781540.

10. **Enhanced postprandial gastric myoelectrical activity after moderate-intensity exercise**. Lu CL, Shidler N, Chen JD. Am J Gastroenterol. 2000 Feb; 95(2): 425-31. PMID: 10685745.

11. **Effects of dietary composition and exercise timing on substrate utilization and sympathoadrenal function in healthy young women**. Matsuo T, Suzuki M. Metabolism. 1999 Dec; 48(12): 1596-602. PMID: 10599994.

12. **Effect of beverage osmolality on intestinal fluid absorption during exercise**. Gisolfi CV, Summers RW, Lambert GP, Xia T. Journal of Applied Physiology. 1998; 85(5): 1941-8. SportDiscus: SPHS-18831.

13. **Effect of hypohydration on gastric emptying and intestinal absorption during exercise**. Ryan AJ, Lambert GP, Shi X, Chang RT, Summers RW, Gisolfi CV. Journal of Applied Physiology. 1998; 84(5): 1581-8. SportDiscus: SPH462902.

14. **Absorption from different intestinal segments during exercise**. Lambert GP, Chang RT, Xia T, Summers RW, Gisolfi CV. Journal of Applied Physiology. 1997; 83(1): 204-12. SportDiscus: SPH419935.

(k) XI. Caffeine and Energy-Drinks

1. **QTc interval prolongation with high dose energy drink consumption in a healthy volunteer**. Shah SA, Lacey CS, Bergendahl T, Kolasa M, Riddock

IC. Int J Cardiol. 2014 Mar 15; 172(2): e336-7. PMID: 24447738.

2. **Methodological and metabolic considerations in the study of caffeine-containing energy drinks**. Shearer J. Nutrition Reviews. 2014; 72: 137-45. SportDiscus: 98716272.

3. **Effects of energy drink major bioactive compounds on the performance of young adults in fitness and cognitive tests: a randomized controlled trial**. Kammerer M, Jaramillo JA, García A, Calderón JC, Valbuena LH. Journal of the International Society of Sports Nutrition. 2014; 11(1): 1-14. SportDiscus: 99363530.

4. **Overuse of energy drinks: why death?** Sanaei-Zadeh H. Am J Emerg Med. 2013 Dec; 31(12): 1713-4. PMID: 24139997.

5. **Death of a young man after overuse of energy drink**. Avci S, Sarikaya R, Buyukcam F. Am J Emerg Med. 2013 Nov; 31(11): 1624 e3-4. PMID: 23896014.

6. **An analysis of energy-drink toxicity in the National Poison Data System**. Seifert SM, Seifert SA, Schaechter JL, Bronstein AC, Benson BE, Hershorin ER, Arheart KL, Franco VI, Lipshultz SE. Clin Toxicol (Phila). 2013 Aug; 51(7): 566-74. PMID: 23879181.

7. **Do the non-caffeine ingredients of energy drinks affect metabolic responses to heavy exercise?** Pettitt RW, Niemeyer JD, Sexton PJ, Lipetzky A, Murray SR. J Strength Cond Res. 2013 Jul; 27(7): 1994-9. PMID: 23037611.

8. **Consumption of energy drinks: a new**

provocation test for primary arrhythmogenic diseases? Gray B, Das KJ, Semsarian C. Int J Cardiol. 2012 Aug 9; 159(1): 77-8. PMID: 22704863.

9. **It took a RedBull to unmask Brugada syndrome**. Rutledge M, Witthed A, Khouzam RN. Int J Cardiol. 2012 Nov 1; 161(1): e14-5. PMID: 22465350.

10. **Reverse Takotsubo cardiomyopathy associated with the consumption of an energy drink**. Kaoukis A, Panagopoulou V, Mojibian HR, Jacoby D. Circulation. 2012 Mar 27; 125(12): 1584-5. PMID: 22451608.

11. **Left main coronary artery acute thrombosis related to energy drink intake**. Benjo AM, Pineda AM, Nascimento FO, Zamora C, Lamas GA, Escolar E. Circulation. 2012 Mar 20; 125(11): 1447-8. PMID: 22431887.

12. **Congenital type 1 long QT syndrome unmasked by a highly caffeinated energy drink**. Dufendach KA, Horner JM, Cannon BC, Ackerman MJ. Heart Rhythm. 2012 Feb; 9(2): 285-8. PMID: 22001708.

13. **Energy Drinks: Ergolytic or Ergogenic?** Sillivent J, Blevins J, Peak K. International Journal of Exercise Science. 2012; 5(3): 214-22. SportDiscus: 82217724.

14. **Myocardial infarction in a young adult following the consumption of a caffeinated energy drink**. Scott MJ, El-Hassan M, Khan AA. BMJ Case Rep. 2011; 2011. PMID: 22693185.

15. **Effects of XS Energy Drink on Aerobic Exercise Capacity of Athletes**. Sheehan KM, Hartzler

LK. International Journal of Exercise Science. 2011; 4(2): 152-63. SportDiscus: 61345792.

16. **Efficacy of pre exercise carbohydrate drink (Gatorade) on the recovery heart rate, blood lactate, and glucose levels in short term intensive exercise.** Singh A, Chaudhary S, Sandhu JS. Serbian Journal of Sports Sciences. 2011; 5(1): 29-34. SportDiscus: 66385377.

17. **The acute effects of two energy drinks on endurance performance in female athlete students.** Kazemi F, Gaeini A, Kordi M, Rahnama N. Sport Sciences for Health. 2010; 5(2): 55-6. SportDiscus: 62290726.

18. **Influence of energy drinks and alcohol on post-exercise heart rate recovery and heart rate variability.** Wiklund U, Karlsson M, Öström M, Messner T. Clinical Physiology & Functional Imaging. 2009; 29(1): 74-80. SportDiscus: 35867631.

19. **Awareness and Use of Caffeine by Athletes Competing at the 2005 Ironman Triathlon World Championships.** Desbrow B, Leveritt M. International Journal of Sport Nutrition & Exercise Metabolism. 2006; 16(5): 545-58. SportDiscus: 23221198.

20. **Caffeine increases exogenous carbohydrate oxidation during exercise.** Yeo SE, Jentjens RLPG, Wallis GA, Jeukendrup AE. Journal of Applied Physiology. 2005; 99(3): 844-50. SportDiscus: 18124319.

21. **The Effect of Two Sports Drinks and Water on GI Complaints and Performance During an 18-km Run.** van Nieuwenhovern MA, Brouns F, Kovacs

EMR. International Journal of Sports Medicine. 2005; 26(4): 281-5. SportDiscus: SPHS-996883.

22. **Effects of a sports nutrition bar on endurance running performance**. Oliver SK, Tremblay MS. Journal of Strength & Conditioning Research (Allen Press Publishing Services Inc.). 2002; 16(1): 152-6. SportDiscus: SPHS-813468.

23. **Gastrointestinal permeability during exercise: effects of aspirin and energy-containing beverages.** Lambert GP, Broussard LJ, Mason BL, Mauermann WJ, Gisolfi CV. Journal of Applied Physiology. 2001; 90(6): 2075-80. SportDiscus: SPHS-781408.

24. **Gastrointestinal function during exercise: comparison of water, sports drink, and sports drink with caffeine.** Van Nieuwenhoven MA, Brummer RM, Brouns F. Journal of Applied Physiology. 2000; 89(3): 1079-85. SportDiscus: SPHS-661215.

25. **Caffeine ingestion and performance of a 1,500-metre swim**. MacIntosh BR, Wright BM. Canadian Journal of Applied Physiology. 1995; 20(2): 168-77. SportDiscus: SPH377662.

26. **Benefits of caffeine ingestion on sprint performance in trained and untrained swimmers**. Collomp K, Ahmaidi S, Chatard JC, Audran M, Prefaut C. European Journal of Applied Physiology & Occupational Physiology. 1992; 64(4): 377-80. SportDiscus: SPH299838.

27. **The metabolic and performance effects of caffeine compared to coffee during endurance**

exercise. Hodgson AB, Randell RK, Jeukendrup AE. PLoS One. 2013; 8(4): e59561. PMID: 23573201.

28. **Caffeine ingestion and performance of a 1,500-metre swim**. MacIntosh BR, Wright BM. Can J Appl Physiol. 1995 Jun; 20(2): 168-77. PMID: 7640644.

(I) XII. Neurological Issues: Autonomic Nervous System and Swimming or Exercise

1. **Autonomic modulation and its relation with body composition in swimmers**. Rossi FE, Ricci-Vitor AL, Sabino JP, Vanderlei LC, Freitas IF, Jr. J Strength Cond Res. 2014 Jul; 28(7): 2047-53.

2. **Evidence of parasympathetic hyperactivity in functionally overreached athletes**. Le Meur Y, Pichon A, Schaal K, Schmitt L, Louis J, Gueneron J, Vidal PP, Hausswirth C. Med Sci Sports Exerc. 2013 Nov; 45(11): 2061-71. PMID: 24136138.

3. **A model for the training effects in swimming demonstrates a strong relationship between parasympathetic activity, performance and index of fatigue**. Chalencon S, Busso T, Lacour JR, Garet M, Pichot V, Connes P, Gabel CP, Roche F, Barthelemy JC. PLoS One. 2012; 7(12): e52636. PMID: 23285121.

4. **Non-invasive measures of cardiac autonomic control following high intensity exercise in endurance trained older male cyclists**. Brown SJ, Ryan H, Brown JA. New Zealand Journal of Sports Medicine. 2007 Summer2007; 35(1): 28-34. SportDiscus: 32577295.

5. **Sympathoadrenergic regulation & the**

adrenoceptor system. Jost J, Weiss M, Weicker H. J Appl Physiol (1985). 1990 Mar; 68(3): 897-904.

6. **Autonomic nervous control of postprandial hemodynamic changes at rest and upright exercise**. Kelbaek H, Munck O, Christensen NJ. Journal of Applied Physiology. 1987; 63(5): 1862-5. SportDiscus: SPH209268.

7. **Sympathoadrenergic regulation**. Weicker H. Int J Sports Med. 1986 Jun; 7 Suppl 1: 16-26.PMID: 3017874.

8. **Autonomic neuroendocrine responses to exercises**. Galbo H. Scandinavian Journal of Sports Sciences. 1986; 6(1): 3-17. SportDiscus: SPH186735.

9. **'Autonomic conflict': a different way to die during cold water immersion?** Michael J Shattock and Michael J Tipton. J Physiol. 2012 Jul 15; 590(Pt 14): 3219–3230. Published online 2012 Apr 30. doi: 10.1113/jphysiol.2012.229864 PMCID: PMC3459038 PMID: 22547634

(m) XIII. Anxiety, Mental Preparation and Performance

1. **Triathlon: how to mentally prepare for the big race**. Bales J, Bales K. Sports Med Arthrosc. 2012 Dec; 20(4): 217-9. PMID: 23147092.

2. **Cognition and performance: anxiety, mood and perceived exertion among Ironman triathletes**. Parry D, Chinnasamy C, Papadopoulou E, Noakes T, Micklewright D. Br J Sports Med. 2011 Nov; 45(14):

1088-94. PMID: 20542977.

3. **Directional anxiety responses in elite and sub-elite young athletes: intensity of anxiety symptoms matters**. Lundqvist C, Kentta G, Raglin JS. Scand J Med Sci Sports. 2011 Dec; 21(6): 853-62. PMID: 22126716.

4. **Heart-rate variability and precompetitive anxiety in swimmers**. Cervantes Blasquez JC, Rodas Font G, Capdevila Ortis L. Psicothema. 2009 Nov; 21(4): 531-6.PMID: 19861094.

5. **Functional impact of emotions on athletic performance: comparing the IZOF model and the directional perception approach**. Robazza C, Pellizzari M, Bertollo M, Hanin YL. J Sports Sci. 2008 Aug; 26(10): 1033-47. PMID: 18608828.

6. **Precompetitive state anxiety, objective and subjective performance, and causal attributions in competitive swimmers**. Polman R, Rowcliffe N, Borkoles E, Levy A. Pediatr Exerc Sci. 2007 Feb; 19(1): 39-50. PMID: 17554156.

7. **Modelling the relationships between training, anxiety, and fatigue in elite athletes**. Millet GP, Groslambert A, Barbier B, Rouillon JD, Candau RB. Int J Sports Med. 2005 Jul-Aug; 26(6): 492-8.PMID: 16037894.

8. **Perceived control of anxiety and its relationship to self-confidence and performance**. Hanton S, Connaughton D. Res Q Exerc Sport. 2002 Mar;73(1):87-97.PMID: 11926488.

9. **Pre-competitive feeling states and directional anxiety interpretations**. Jones G, Hanton S. J Sports Sci. 2001 Jun; 19(6): 385-95. PMID: 11411775.

10. **Competitive worries, sport confidence, and performance ratings for young swimmers**. Psychountaki M, Zervas Y. Percept Mot Skills. 2000 Aug; 91(1): 87-94. PMID: 11011876.

11. **Antecedents of intensity and direction dimensions of competitive anxiety as a function of skill**. Hanton S, Jones G. Psychol Rep. 1997 Dec; 81(3 Pt 2): 1139-47. PMID: 9461747.

12. **Path analysis examining relationships among antecedents of anxiety, multidimensional state anxiety, and triathlon performance**. Lane AM, Terry PC, Karageorghis CI. Percept Mot Skills. 1995 Dec; 81(3 Pt 2): 1255-66. PMID: 8684922.

13. **Changes in mood states during training in female and male college swimmers**. Raglin JS, Morgan WP, O'Connor PJ. Int J Sports Med. 1991 Dec; 12(6): 585-9. PMID: 1797703.

14. **Pre-competition anxiety and performance in female high school swimmers: a test of optimal function theory**. Raglin JS, Morgan WP, Wise KJ. Int J Sports Med. 1990 Jun; 11(3): 171-5. PMID: 2373573.

15. **Collegiate swimmers: sex differences in self-reports and indices of physiological stress**. Gackenbach J. Percept Mot Skills. 1982 Oct; 55(2): 555-8. PMID: 7155753.

16. **Anxiety and the competitive swimmer**. Hogg JM. Can J Appl Sport Sci. 1980 Sep; 5(3): 183-7. PMID: 7004656.

XIV. Cardiac Issues: Sudden Cardiac Death

in Swimming

1. **Sudden cardiac death during open water swimming**. Tipton MJ. Br J Sports Med. 2014 Aug; 48(15): 1134-5.PMID: 23377278.

2. **Characteristics and outcomes of sudden cardiac arrest during sports in women**. Marijon E, Bougouin W, Celermajer DS, Perier MC, Dumas F, Benameur N, Karam N, Lamhaut L, Tafflet M, Mustafic H, et al. Circ Arrhythm Electrophysiol. 2013 Dec; 6(6): 1185-91. PMID: 24190898.

3. **Unexpected sudden death due to recreational swimming and diving in men in Croatia in a 14-year period**. Durakovic Z, Durakovic MM, Skavic J, Gojanovic MD. Coll Antropol. 2012 Jun; 36(2): 641-5. PMID: 22856257.

4. **Cardiovascular damage resulting from chronic excessive endurance exercise**. Patil HR, O'Keefe JH, Lavie CJ, Magalski A, Vogel RA, McCullough PA. Mo Med. 2012 Jul-Aug; 109(4): 312-21.PMID: 22953596.

5. **Sudden cardiac death in a 20-year-old male swimmer**. Cedrone AJ, Makaryus JN, Catanzaro JN, Ruisi P, Romich TJ, Horan P, Makaryus AN, Jauhar S. South Med J. 2010 May; 103(5): 464-6. PMID: 20375931.

6. **Electrocardiographic amplitudes: a new risk factor for sudden death in hypertrophic cardiomyopathy**. Ostman-Smith I, Wisten A, Nylander E, Bratt EL, Granelli A, Oulhaj A, Ljungstrom E. Eur Heart J. 2010 Feb; 31(4): 439-49. PMID: 19897498.

7. **Causes of sudden death during**

the triathlon. Constantini NW, Dubnov-Raz G, Mountjoy M. JAMA. 2010 Jul 21; 304(3): 269; author reply -70.PMID: 20639556.

8. **Sudden death during the triathlon.** Harris KM, Henry JT, Rohman E, Haas TS, Maron BJ. JAMA. 2010 Apr 7; 303(13): 1255-7.PMID: 20371783.

9. **T-wave variability detects abnormalities in ventricular repolarization: a prospective study comparing healthy persons and Olympic athletes.** Heinz L, Sax A, Robert F, Urhausen A, Balta O, Kreuz J, Nickenig G, Ocklenburg R, Schwab JO. Ann Noninvasive Electrocardiol. 2009 Jul; 14(3): 276-9. PMID: 19614640.

10. **Images in cardiovascular medicine. Sudden cardiac death due to triple vessel coronary dissection.** Lunebourg A, Letovanec I, Eggenberger P, Lehr HA. Circulation. 2008 Apr 15; 117(15): 2038-40. PMID: 18413511.

11. **The upper limit of physiological cardiac hypertrophy in elite male and female athletes: the British experience.** Whyte GP, George K, Sharma S, Firoozi S, Stephens N, Senior R, McKenna WJ. Eur J Appl Physiol. 2004 Aug; 92(4-5): 592-7. PMID: 15054661.

12. **Effects of half ironman competition on the development of late potentials.** Warburton DER, Welsh RC, Haykowsky MJ, Taylor DA, Humen DP, Dzavik V. Med Sci Sports Exerc. 2000 Jul; 32(7): 1208-13. PMID: 10912883.

13. **Physiological or pseudophysiological ECG**

changes in endurance-trained athletes. Claessens P, Claessens C, Claessens M, Henderieckx J, Claessens J. Heart Vessels. 2000; 15(4): 181-90. PMID: 11471658.

14. Ventricular premature beats in triathletes: still a physiological phenomenon? Claessens P, Claessens C, Claessens M, Bloemen H, Verbanck M, Fagard R. Cardiology. 1999; 92(1): 28-38. PMID: 10640794.

15. Is hyperkalaemia the cause of sudden death in young healthy athletes? Busuttil A. Med Sci Law. 1990 Oct; 30(4): 341-4. PMID: 2263180.

16. Swimming and loss of consciousness. Suzuki T, Ikeda N, Umetsu K, Kashimura S. Z Rechtsmed. 1985; 94(2): 121-6. PMID: 4002881.

17. Sudden death of a champion athlete. Autopsy findings. Noakes TD, Rose AG, Benjamin J. S Afr Med J. 1984 Sep 22; 66(12): 458-9. PMID: 6541373.

18. Sudden swimming deaths: a psychomotor reinterpretation. Binik YM, Sullivan MJ. Psychophysiology. 1983 Nov; 20(6): 670-81. PMID: 6657856.

19. Sudden Death in cold water and ventricular arrhythmia. Keatinge WR, Hayward MG. J Forensic Sci. 1981 Jul; 26(3): 459-61. PMID: 7252459.

20. Cold immersion and swimming. Keatinge WR. J R Nav Med Serv. 1972 Winter; 58(3): 171-6.PMID: 4647866.

(n) XV. Cardiac Arrhythmias

1. **Right ventricular adaptations and arrhythmias in amateur ultra-endurance athletes.** Rimensberger C, Carlen F, Brugger N, Seiler C, Wilhelm M. Br J Sports Med. 2014 Aug; 48(15): 1179-84. PMID: 24357641.

2. **A 34-year-old triathlete with hyperthermia.** Jordan K. J Emerg Nurs. 2013 Nov; 39(6): 623-4. PMID: 24054731.

3. **Pulmonary vein stenosis after radiofrequency ablation of lone atrial fibrillation in an ironman triathlete.** Poussel M, Chodek-Hingray A, Mandry D, Fronzaroli E, Netter F, Chenuel B. Int J Cardiol. 2013 Mar 10; 163(3): e39-41. PMID: 23010442.

4. **Potential adverse cardiovascular effects from excessive endurance exercise.** O'Keefe JH, Patil HR, Lavie CJ, Magalski A, Vogel RA, McCullough PA. Mayo Clin Proc. 2012 Jun; 87(6): 587-95. PMID: 22677079.

5. **Breath holding with water immersion in synchronized swimmers and untrained women.** Alentejano TC, Marshall D, Bell GJ. Res Sports Med. 2010 Apr; 18(2): 97-114.PMID: 20397113.

6. **Unraveling the mechanism of a wide-complex tachycardia.** Horduna I, Roy D, Talajic M, Khairy P. J Cardiovasc Electrophysiol. 2009 Jul; 20(7): 823-4. PMID: 19298564.

7. **Exercise-induced right ventricular dysplasia/cardiomyopathy — an emerging condition distinct from arrhythmogenic right ventricular dysplasia/cardiomyopathy.** Harper RW,

Mottram PM. Heart Lung Circ. 2009 Jun; 18(3): 233-5. PMID: 18396459.

8. **Haemodynamic and arrhythmic effects of moderately cold (22 degrees C) water immersion and swimming in patients with stable coronary artery disease and heart failure**. Schmid JP, Morger C, Noveanu M, Binder RK, Anderegg M, Saner H. Eur J Heart Fail. 2009 Sep; 11(9): 903-9. PMID: 19696059.

9. **Apnea-induced changes in time estimation and its relation to bradycardia**. Jamin T, Joulia F, Fontanari P, Giacomoni M, Bonnon M, Vidal F, Cremieux J. Aviat Space Environ Med. 2004

10. **Syncope in a triathlete**. Scott WA. Curr Sports Med Rep. 2003 Jun; 2(3): 157-8. PMID: 12831655.

11. **Identification of patients at risk during swimming by Holter monitoring**. Niebauer J, Hambrecht R, Hauer K, Marburger C, Schoppenthau M, Kalberer B, Schlierf G, Kubler W, Schuler G. Am J Cardiol. 1994 Oct 1; 74(7): 651-6.PMID: 7942521.

12. **Increased heart rate and blood pressure response, and occurrence of arrhythmias in elderly swimmers**. Itoh M, Araki H, Hotokebuchi N, Takeshita T, Gotoh K, Nishi K. J Sports Med Phys Fitness. 1994 Jun; 34(2): 169-78. PMID: 7526043.

13. **Changes in cardiac rhythm in man during underwater submersion and swimming studied by ECG telemetry**. Yamaguchi H, Tanaka H, Obara S, Tanabe S, Utsuyama N, Takahashi A, Nakahira J, Yamamoto Y, Jiang ZL, He J, et al. Eur J Appl Physiol Occup Physiol. 1993; 66(1): 43-8. PMID: 8425511.

14. **Syncope secondary to paroxysmal high grade AV block in a heavily trained man**. Hurwitz JL, Conley MJ, Wharton JM, Prystowsky EN. Pacing Clin Electrophysiol. 1991 Jun; 14(6): 994-9. PMID: 1715076.

15. **The 'athletic heart syndrome'. A critical review**. George KP, Wolfe LA, Burggraf GW. Sports Med. 1991 May; 11(5): 300-30.PMID: 1829849.

16. **Cardiac output and heart rate in man during simulated swimming while breath-holding**. Paulev PE, Pokorski M, Honda Y, Morikawa T, Sakakibara Y, Tanaka Y. Jpn J Physiol. 1990; 40(1): 117-25. PMID: 2362379.

17. **Heart rate in humans during underwater swimming with and without breath-hold**. Butler PJ, Woakes AJ. Respir Physiol. 1987 Sep; 69(3): 387-99. PMID: 3659605.

18. **Heart rate and rhythm during underwater swimming**. Jakopin J, Rakovec P. Cardiologia. 1982; 27(2): 205-10.PMID: 6927433.

19. **Behavior of heart rate and incidence of arrhythmia in swimming and diving**. Jung K, Stolle W. Biotelem Patient Monit. 1981; 8(4): 228-39. PMID: 7337825.

20. **Letter: Collapse during channel swim**. Keatingewr. Lancet. 1976 Sep 25; 2(7987): 692. PMID: 60554.

21. **Wenckebach A-V block: a frequent feature following heavy physical training**. Meytes I, Kaplinsky E, Yahini JH, Hanne-Paparo N, Neufeld HN. Am Heart

J. 1975 Oct; 90(4): 426-30. PMID: 1163436.

22. **Death as an expression of functional disease**. Pruitt RD. Mayo Clin Proc. 1974 Sep; 49(9): 627-34. PMID: 4606407.

23. **Underwater bradycardia**. Burke EJ, Jr., Lynch PR. J Sports Med. 1974 May-Jun; 2(3): 163-6. PMID: 4468330.

24. **Electrocardiogram of the athlete. Alterations simulating those of organic heart disease**. Lichtman J, O'Rourke RA, Klein A, Karliner JS. Arch Intern Med. 1973 Nov; 132(5): 763-70.PMID: 4270763.

25. **The electrocardiogram in swimmers**. Jenkins DH, MacLeod A, MacKay S. J Sports Med Phys Fitness. 1972 Dec; 12(7): 246-9.PMID: 4669141.

26. **Man's responses to breath-hold exercise in air and in water**. Craig AB, Jr., Medd WL. J Appl Physiol. 1968 Jun; 24(6): 773-7. PMID: 5653161.

27. **Seasonal observations on the cardiac rhythm during diving in the Korean ama**. Hong SK, Song SH, Kim PK, Suh CS. J Appl Physiol. 1967 Jul; 23(1): 18-22. PMID: 6028157.

(o) XVI. Long QT Syndrome

1. **Unexplained drownings and the cardiac channelopathies: a molecular autopsy series**. Tester DJ, Medeiros-Domingo A, Will ML, Ackerman MJ. Mayo Clin Proc. 2011 Oct; 86(10): 941-7. PMID: 21964171.

2. **Presentation and outcome of water-related events in children with long QT syndrome**. Albertella

L, Crawford J, Skinner JR. Arch Dis Child. 2011
Aug;96(8):704-7. PMID: 21131640.

3. **Spectrum and frequency of cardiac channel
defects in swimming-triggered arrhythmia
syndromes**. Choi G, Kopplin LJ, Tester DJ, Will ML,
Haglund CM, Ackerman MJ. Circulation. 2004 Oct 12;
110(15): 2119-24. PMID: 15466642.

4. **Who is at risk for cardiac events in young
patients with long QT syndrome?** Yoshinaga M,
Nagashima M, Shibata T, Niimura I, Kitada M, Yasuda T,
Iwamoto M, Kamimura J, Iino M, Horigome H, et al.
Circ J. 2003 Dec; 67(12): 1007-12. PMID: 14639015.

5. **Images in cardiovascular medicine.
Ventricular fibrillation during swimming in a patient
with long-QT syndrome**. Ott P, Marcus FI, Moss AJ.
Circulation. 2002 Jul 23; 106(4): 521-2. PMID: 12135956.

6. **Mechanism of sudden cardiac arrest
while swimming in a child with the prolonged QT
syndrome**. Batra AS, Silka MJ. J Pediatr. 2002 Aug;
141(2): 283-4. PMID: 12183730.

7. **Comparison of clinical and genetic variables
of cardiac events associated with loud noise
versus swimming among subjects with the long QT
syndrome**. Moss AJ, Robinson JL, Gessman L, Gillespie
R, Zareba W, Schwartz PJ, Vincent GM, Benhorin J,
Heilbron EL, Towbin JA, et al. Am J Cardiol. 1999 Oct
15; 84(8): 876-9. PMID: 10532503.

8. **Face immersion in cold water induces
prolongation of the QT interval and T-wave changes
in children with nonfamilial long QT syndrome**.

Yoshinaga M, Kamimura J, Fukushige T, Kusubae R, Shimago A, Nishi J, Kono Y, Nomura Y, Miyata K. Am J Cardiol. 1999 May 15; 83(10): 1494-7, A8. PMID: 10335770.

9. **Swimming, a gene-specific arrhythmogenic trigger for inherited long QT syndrome**. Ackerman MJ, Tester DJ, Porter CJ. Mayo Clin Proc. 1999 Nov; 74(11): 1088-94. PMID: 10560595.

10. **Identification of a family with inherited long QT syndrome after a pediatric near-drowning**. Ackerman MJ, Porter CJ. Pediatrics. 1998 Feb; 101(2): 306-8. PMID: 9445509.

(p) XVII. Heart Diseases

1. **The mystery of swimming deaths in athletes**. Eichner ER. Curr Sports Med Rep. 2011 Jan-Feb; 10(1): 3-4. PMID: 21228643.

2. **Remote preconditioning improves maximal performance in highly trained athletes**. Jean-St-Michel E, Manlhiot C, Li J, Tropak M, Michelsen MM, Schmidt MR, McCrindle BW, Wells GD, Redington AN. Med Sci Sports Exerc. 2011 Jul;43(7):1280-6. PMID: 21131871.

3. **By the way, doctor. When I attempt to go into the outdoor pool at my beach club, I gasp for breath, get dizzy and light-headed, and have to get out. Several years ago, I read an article that some people who are very sensitive to cold water may sustain a heart attack from submersion into cold water. Is this a possibility?** Lee TH. Harv Health Lett. 2010 May;

35(7): 4. PMID: 20589961.

4. **Myocardial contrast echocardiography for the distinction of hypertrophic cardiomyopathy from athlete's heart and hypertensive heart disease**. Indermuhle A, Vogel R, Rutz T, Meier P, Seiler C. Swiss Med Wkly. 2009 Nov 28; 139(47-48): 691-8. PMID: 20047131.

5. **Alteration in left ventricular strains and torsional mechanics after ultralong duration exercise in athletes**. Nottin S, Doucende G, Schuster I, Tanguy S, Dauzat M, Obert P. Circ Cardiovasc Imaging. 2009 Jul; 2(4): 323-30. PMID: 19808613.

6. **Biochemical and functional abnormalities of left and right ventricular function after ultra-endurance exercise**. La Gerche A, Connelly KA, Mooney DJ, MacIsaac AI, Prior DL. Heart. 2008 Jul; 94(7): 860-6.PMID: 17483127.

7. **Treat the patient not the blood test: the implications of an increase in cardiac troponin after prolonged endurance exercise**. Whyte G, Stephens N, Senior R, George K, Shave R, Wilson M, Sharma S. Br J Sports Med. 2007 Sep; 41(9): 613-5; discussion 5. PMID: 17261549.

8. **Atrioventricular plane displacement is the major contributor to left ventricular pumping in healthy adults, athletes, and patients with dilated cardiomyopathy**. Carlsson M, Ugander M, Mosen H, Buhre T, Arheden H. Am J Physiol Heart Circ Physiol. 2007 Mar; 292(3): H1452-9. PMID: 17098822.

9. **Arterial blood pressure analysis based on**

scattering transform II. Laleg TM, Medigue C, Cottin F, Sorine M. Conf Proc IEEE Eng Med Biol Soc. 2007; 2007: 5330-3.PMID: 18003211.

10. **Left ventricular dysfunction and chronic heart failure: should aqua therapy and swimming be allowed?** Meyer K. Br J Sports Med. 2006 Oct; 40(10): 817-8. PMID: 16990443.

11. **The relative myocardial blood volume differentiates between hypertensive heart disease and athlete's heart in humans**. Indermuhle A, Vogel R, Meier P, Wirth S, Stoop R, Mohaupt MG, Seiler C. Eur Heart J. 2006 Jul; 27(13): 1571-8. PMID: 16717078.

12. **Raised troponin T and echocardiographic abnormalities after prolonged strenuous exercise—the Australian Ironman Triathlon**. Tulloh L, Robinson D, Patel A, Ware A, Prendergast C, Sullivan D, Pressley L. Br J Sports Med. 2006 Jul; 40(7): 605-9. PMID: 16611724.

13. **Sex-specific characteristics of cardiac function, geometry, and mass in young adult elite athletes**. Petersen SE, Hudsmith LE, Robson MD, Doll HA, Francis JM, Wiesmann F, Jung BA, Hennig J, Watkins H, Neubauer S. J Magn Reson Imaging. 2006 Aug; 24(2): 297-303.PMID: 16823779.

(q) XVIII. Wetsuit and Buoyancy Effects in Open Water Swimming.

1.Wetsuits, body density and swimming performance. L Cordain and R Kopriva Br J Sports

Med. 1991 Mar; 25(1): 31–33. PMID: 1913028
http://www.ncbi.nlm.nih.gov/pmc/articles/PMC147880
3/?page=1

2.Swimming performances in long distance open-water events with and without wetsuit.
Ulsamer S1, Rüst CA1, Rosemann T1, Lepers R2, Knechtle B3.
BMC Sports Sci Med Rehabil. 2014 May 21; 6: 20. doi: 10.1186/2052-1847-6-20. eCollection 2014.

3. Wet suit effect: a comparison between competitive swimmers and triathletes. Chatard JC1, Senegas X, Selles M, Dreanot P, Geyssant A. Med Sci Sports Exerc. 1995 Apr; 27(4): 580-6.

Open Access J Sports Med

4.The relationship of wearing a wetsuit in long-distance open-water swimming with sex, age, calendar year, performance, and nationality – crossing the "Strait of Gibraltar"
Pantelis Theodoros Nikolaidis, Caio Victor Sousa, and Beat Knechtle. 2018; 9: 27–36.

Published online 2018 Feb 21. doi: 10.2147/OAJSM.S158502
PMCID: PMC5825996
PMID: 29503588

5. Human body buoyancy: a study of 98 men. Donoghue ER, Minnigerode SC. J Forensic Sci. 1977 Jul; 22(3): 573-9.

PART 5: Appendix

Acknowledgements.

Although this book is a reflection of my passion for open water swimming, it was inspired by many who shared with me their own passions and experiences in open water.

On a personal level, after many years of watching my wife Dale swim endless lengths (seemingly effortlessly), and then watching our children start doing the same, I was inspired to personally dig deep and get humble to finally face a lifetime angst, and learn how to swim—enough to even enjoy it. After a few "Eureka!" moments, my passions for learning swimming in open water began shortly after that, as did the fascination and desire to document the necessary progression through the unique skills required for open water swimming. Essentially, I have enjoyed becoming a student of my own experience, so that I could share it with readers like you. It has been fun for me expand my open water horizons, especially because I hope this *"Swimming In Open Water"* series can also help you.

Here in Kelowna, British Columbia, where Canada's largest open water swim event (the Across The Lake Swim) has continued uninterrupted since 1949, it is clear that tireless efforts have nurtured this event over many decades by coaches and volunteers alike; their dedication has perpetuated an undeniably infectious enthusiasm for sharing open water swimming skills, helping so many people to reach one of their bucket list goals—swimming across Lake Okanagan-- including me. In recent years, more than 1000 swimmers have signed up for the event, almost half of them for the first time. If you have a similar love for open water swimming, I invite you to come join us each July (see more at www.acrossthelakeswim.com). The event is now ranked as one of the Top 100 Open Water Swims in The World.

About the Author.

Mark Fromberg, M.D. was born and raised in Vancouver, British Columbia, where he completed a B.Sc. in Kinesiology before completing medical school in 1985. Although he retired after 30 years of practice in primary care and urgent care medicine, he remains actively involved in various community preventive health initiatives in Kelowna, B.C., where he has lived and raised a family with his wife for the last 25 years.

Although Dr. Fromberg has participated in a wide variety of competitive sports in his lifetime, he only learned how to swim as 50 year old adult, a process that fostered his interest in open water swimming events and triathlon. After many years as a triathlete, he became a certified triathlon coach, and subsequently has long been involved in medical support of many triathlons, including directing the Ironman Canada medical tent (2010-2012) and the Kelowna Apple Triathlon (2010-2015), along many smaller community events. As part of a team of specialists, he has had the privilege of providing medical services in the Kona Ironman medical tent for many years as well (2008-2014).

Dr. Fromberg has also enjoyed being a director of

Canada's largest open water swim event for more than 10 years, overseeing the 5-fold growth of Kelowna's Across The Lake Swim (ATLS) in that time. This event has developed a unique partnership with the local Y, where the funds raised by the ATLS are used to provide swimming lessons to every grade III and IV child in the region, thereby drown-proofing a generation of kids. The initiative won a Health Promotion Award in 2015 from the Doctors of BC.

The Swimming in Open Water Series

This book is the second of three in the Swimming in Open Water series, which is intended to encapsulate the skills for the development of confidence, enjoyment in open water, while providing the physiological knowledge base to enhance swimming safety in open water. The first book, published in early 2018, has the subtitle, "Become Less Anxious and More Confident When Getting In Over Your Head", and is directed to the beginner swimmer, or those who are transitioning from pool swimming to open water. The third book, scheduled for release in mid 2019, is a race director's guide as to how to put on a safe event that also encourages growth and interest in open water swimming, while secretly stimulating a local population's commitment to a lifetime of health and fitness in a sport that you can do until you are 100. These books are available on Amazon, in both paperback and eBook versions.

Made in the USA
Columbia, SC
18 September 2023